Orthopaedic Biomechanics Made Easy

Sheraz S. Malik, MRCS, MSc
trust-grade registrar in orthopaedics, Newham University Hospital, Barts Healthcare
NHS Trust, UK

Shahbaz S. Malik, MRCS, MSc
specialty registrar in orthopaedics, West Midlands Deanery, UK

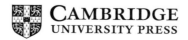
CAMBRIDGE
UNIVERSITY PRESS

CAMBRIDGE
UNIVERSITY PRESS

University Printing House, Cambridge CB2 8BS, United Kingdom

Cambridge University Press is part of the University of Cambridge.

It furthers the University's mission by disseminating knowledge in the pursuit of education, learning and research at the highest international levels of excellence.

www.cambridge.org
Information on this title: www.cambridge.org/9781107685468

© Sheraz S. Malik and Shahbaz S. Malik 2015

First published 2015

Printed in the United Kingdom by TJ International Ltd. Padstow Cornwall

A catalogue record for this publication is available from the British Library

Library of Congress Cataloguing in Publication data
Malik, Sheraz S., author.
Orthopaedic biomechanics made easy / Sheraz S. Malik, Shahbaz S. Malik.
    p. ; cm.
Includes bibliographical references and index.
ISBN 978-1-107-68546-8 (Paperback)
I. Malik, Shahbaz S., author.   II. Title.
[DNLM: 1. Musculoskeletal Physiological Phenomena.
2. Orthopedics–physiology.   3. Biomechanical Phenomena. WE 102]
QP303
612.7′6–dc23   2014021240

ISBN 978-1-107-68546-8 Paperback

To our parents Muhammad S. Malik and Shahnaz Akhtar for their prayers and blessings, and showing us the value of education whether being taught or teaching others, and to our brother, Shahzad S. Malik, for being there for us.

Sheraz S. Malik

Also to my wife Nadia, for her endless patience.

Shahbaz S. Malik

CONTENTS

Part I: Orthopaedic biomaterials and their properties

Part II: Engineering theory applied to orthopaedics

Part III: Clinical biomechanics

CONTENTS

CONTRIBUTORS

Usman Ahmed MRCS, PhD
Specialty Registrar in Trauma & Orthopaedics
West Midlands Deanery

Bola Akinola MRCS, MSc, FRCS (Tr & Orth)
Specialty Registrar in Trauma & Orthopaedics
East of England Deanery

Chee Gan FRCR
Interventional Neuroradiology Fellow
The National Hospital of Neurology and Neurosurgery

Simon MacLean MRCS(Ed) FRCS (Tr & Orth)
Specialty Registrar in Trauma & Orthopaedics
West Midlands Deanery

Ravi Shenoy MRCS(Ed), MS(Orth), DNB(Orth), MD
Specialty Registrar in Trauma & Orthopaedics
Northeast (Stanmore) Rotation, London Deanery

Proofreading and editing work
By
Pritam Tharmarajah MRSC(Ed), MD
Specialty Registrar in General Practice
East Midlands Deanery

Art direction and illustrations
By
Shaheryar Malik

This type of surgery demands training in mechanical techniques, which, though elementary in practical engineering, are as yet unknown in the training of a surgeon.

Sir John Charnley

Everything should be made as simple as possible, but no simpler.

Albert Einstein

PREFACE

Orthopaedic Biomechanics Made Easy introduces you to the fundamental biomechanical principles in orthopaedics, and shows you how these relate to the clinical practice. The book seeks to fulfil two objectives:

- To bring together important biomechanical concepts relevant to surgical practice.
- To make these ideas simple and easy to learn.

Our efforts have been about taking you back to the first principles, and making them more interesting and fun to learn. We have avoided point-by-point references for this reason, as we feel that this might affect the reading experience.

To help you explore the subject, the book is signposted into three parts: Orthopaedic biomaterials and their properties; Engineering theory applied to orthopaedics; and, Clinical biomechanics. Each concept is introduced and explained in a discrete double-page spread. Consecutive sections are usually related and follow a common theme. Naturally, some ideas are more difficult than others, and we expect you to skip over them initially and to come back to them after covering the simpler topics. You do not need to deal with advanced maths to understand the presented biomechanical principles. Mathematical explanations are provided in some sections only to demonstrate how a particular biomechanical fact is derived. You may skip over the mathematical workings without missing out on the learning points.

We hope this book helps to make your clinical practice easier and more rewarding.

Sheraz S. Malik
Shahbaz S. Malik

ACKNOWLEDGEMENTS

We are grateful to Miss Caroline Hing at St George's Healthcare NHS Trust for advice and help in setting up this project. We are in debt to two groups of teachers: the faculty at Cardiff School of Engineering, Cardiff University, where we read MSc in Orthopaedic Engineering, and our clinical trainers for sharing their experience and wisdom. Thanks also to our colleagues at the Engineering School and various hospitals for the group discussions that helped to clarify and develop ideas.

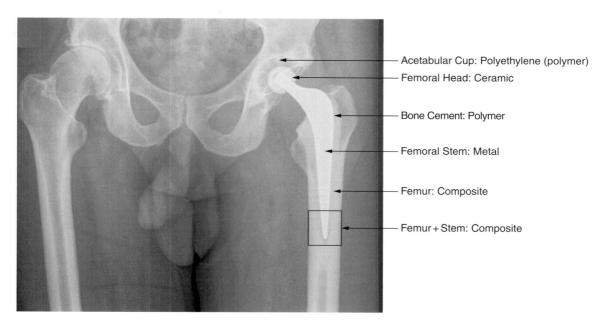

Acetabular Cup: Polyethylene (polymer)
Femoral Head: Ceramic
Bone Cement: Polymer
Femoral Stem: Metal
Femur: Composite
Femur + Stem: Composite

Just as there are three states of matter: solid, liquid and gas, there are three basic forms of solid materials: metals, ceramics and polymers. A composite is formed when any of the types of materials combine in an insoluble state. This radiograph shows all four types of solid material in function in a total hip replacement. The internal structure of the materials produces their unique physical properties, which are utilised in designing orthopaedic implants.

Introduction to orthopaedic biomechanics

Orthopaedic surgery is the branch of medicine that deals with congenital and developmental, degenerative and traumatic conditions of the musculoskeletal system. Mechanics is the science concerned with loads acting on physical bodies and the effects produced by these loads. Biomechanics is the application of mechanics to biological systems. Therefore, orthopaedic biomechanics is about the effects of loads acting on the musculoskeletal system only or with the associated orthopaedic interventions.

Mechanics, and therefore biomechanics, is divided into two main domains:

- *Statics* is concerned with the effects of loads without reference to time. Static analysis is applied when the body is stationary or at one instant in time during dynamic activity.
- *Dynamics* addresses the effects of loads over time. It is further divided into two main subjects:
  - *Kinematics* describes motion of a body over time and includes analyses such as displacement, velocity and acceleration.
  - *Kinetics* is the study of forces associated with the motion of a body.

The main functions of the musculoskeletal system are to support loads and to provide motion of body segments. These two functions come together to achieve the musculoskeletal system's third main purpose: to provide locomotion, i.e. movement from one place to another. These are all mechanical tasks and therefore mechanics can be applied to the musculoskeletal system in the same way as to ordinary mechanical systems. Biomechanics is, in fact, a fundamental basis of orthopaedic practice: the mechanics of the body guide the principles of orthopaedic interventions. Biomechanics is also central to the design and function of modern orthopaedic devices. The orthopaedic surgeon therefore has the responsibility to understand musculoskeletal biomechanics and materials and structural limitations of orthopaedic devices and the principles of their application in order to minimise failure.

This chapter introduces fundamental biomechanical concepts. It defines different types of loads and material properties, and the relationships between them. All the physical interactions between loads and materials can be considered in terms of the two domains of biomechanics mentioned above: statics and dynamics. This book, in fact, focuses on these basic interactions; the different sections simply consider the fundamental statics, kinematic or kinetic aspects of the musculoskeletal system and/or orthopaedic interventions. The basic principles are introduced and explained in the initial sections, and then integrated together in the latter sections. Therefore, even if the biomechanical concepts become complex, they can always be considered in terms of statics, kinematics and kinetics.

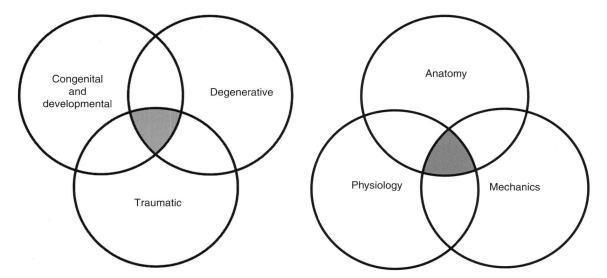

Fig. 1.1 Orthopaedic surgery is the branch of medicine that deals with congenital and developmental, degenerative and traumatic conditions of the musculoskeletal system. Although it is a surgical discipline, over two-thirds of patients with orthopaedic issues are managed with non-surgical treatments.

Fig. 1.2 Biomechanics merges together three sciences: anatomy, physiology and mechanics

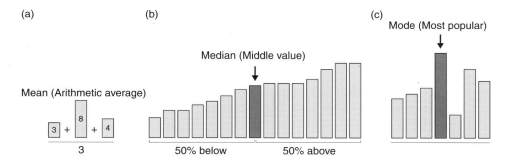

Fig. 1.3 The loads acting on the musculoskeletal system can be considered in the same way as averages in mathematics. The average of a data set can be represented by (a) mean, (b) median or (c) mode – the average that is considered depends on the conditions of the data set. In the same way, loads acting on the musculoskeletal system can be represented by force, stress or strain – the load that is considered depends on the conditions of the loading situation.

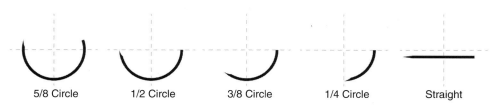

Fig. 1.4 Orthopaedic biomechanics is a fundamental basis of orthopaedic practice. The understanding of biomechanics is as essential in orthopaedics as the understanding of properties of the different types of sutures and needles in surgical practice.

Force

Force is a simple way of representing load in biomechanics. Force is defined as the action of one object on another. Therefore, there must be interaction between two objects to produce a force. Force can have two effects on the object it is acting upon: it can change the shape and/or the state of motion of the object.

Force is a vector quantity, which means that it has a magnitude and a direction. Force, in fact, has three characteristics: magnitude, direction and point of application; and direction is further divided into 'line of action' and 'sense' of the force. All these factors determine the effect of a force on an object. In diagrams, force is drawn as a vector arrow that represents these four characteristics.

When there are multiple forces acting on an object, they can be resolved into a single 'resultant' force that has the same effect as all the other forces acting together. However, forces cannot just be added together, as their direction must also be taken into consideration. A single force can also be broken down into two component forces, which are usually taken perpendicular to each other as 'rectangular' components.

Newton's laws of motion

A force can change the motion of an object. Newton's laws of motion explain the relationship between force and motion:

- *Newton's first law* states that a resultant force must act on an object to change its state of motion. Therefore, a stationary object remains stationary and a moving object maintains its velocity, i.e. speed and direction, unless a resultant force acts on it.

  This law shows that objects have an inherent reluctance to change in their motion. This built-in resistance to change in motion is known as inertia. Inertia is directly proportional to the mass of an object.

- *Newton's second law* states that a resultant force leads to a change in momentum of an object. Therefore, a resultant force causes an object to accelerate (or decelerate).

  This law shows that force is directly proportional to acceleration.

- *Newton's third law* states that, for every force, there is an equal and opposite force. As force is basically an 'action', therefore every action has an equal and opposite reaction.

  This law shows that forces *always* act in pairs and that the two forces are *always* equal in magnitude but opposite in direction. These forces do not simply cancel each other out because they are acting on different objects.

Newton's laws of motion are principles of interaction between different forces and between forces and the material world. These are fundamental to understanding the biomechanics of the musculoskeletal system (Table 1.1).

(a)

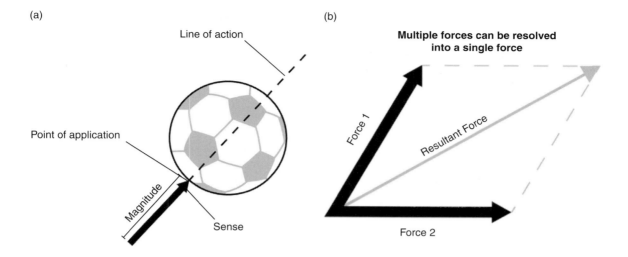

(b)

Multiple forces can be resolved into a single force

(c)

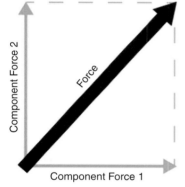

A single force can be broken down into component forces

Fig. 1.5 Force is the action of one object on another. It is drawn as a vector arrow that represents the four characteristics of force: (a) magnitude, point of application, line of action and sense. The displacement of the football is affected by a change in any of these variables. (b) Multiple forces can be resolved into a single force, and (c) a single force can be broken down into component forces, which are usually taken perpendicular to each other as rectangular components.

Table 1.1. **Forces acting on the musculoskeletal system**

Two types of forces act on an object: internal and external forces. Internal forces are the molecular forces found within the object. These are expressed in all directions. Internal forces do not have a specific action on the object, but instead hold it together. Internal forces are considered to be unlimited, but with the overall effect of producing no resultant action on the object. Different components of the musculoskeletal systems, e.g. bones and muscles, all have internal forces acting within them.

External forces are the usual forces that represent the action of one object on another. External forces acting on the musculoskeletal system arise due to *the action of another object on the musculoskeletal system*. External forces are produced in only three ways in the musculoskeletal system:

- action of a part of the body, e.g. muscle contraction
- action of gravity of Earth, i.e. weight
- reaction* from other objects, e.g. the ground.

Joint reaction* force, or joint force, is an unusual internal force. It acts within a joint and holds it together, but its point of application is at the contact point between two bones. Therefore, it acts within a structure, i.e. a joint, as well as between two structures, i.e. bones. As a result, although joint reaction force is an internal force, it can also be considered as an external force. Therefore, the fourth external force considered in the musculoskeletal system analyses is:

- joint reaction force.

* The term 'reaction' in this context simply means 'contact', so a reaction force is due to contact between two objects.

Moment of a force

A force acting on an object can cause it to rotate. This turning effect of a force is called the moment or torque. The moment of a force depends on the magnitude of force and perpendicular distance from the force to the axis (also known as the lever arm):

$$\text{Moment [Nm]} = \text{Force [N]} \times \text{Distance [m]}*$$

Moments are conventionally described as clockwise or anticlockwise.

Couple

A couple is formed when two forces acting on an object are equal in magnitude and opposite in direction, but have different (but parallel) lines of action. A couple produces no resultant force; it only produces a moment on the object.

Conditions of equilibrium

In equilibrium, an object maintains its state of motion, i.e. a stationary object remains stationary and a moving object maintains its velocity. An object is in equilibrium only when:
- there is no resultant force acting on it, i.e. the sum of all forces is zero
- there is no resultant moment acting on it, i.e. the sum of all moments is zero.

This is the application of Newton's first law of motion.

Levers

A lever is a simple machine that operates on moments. It consists of a rigid bar that rotates about an axis, and has two forces acting on it: an applied force that works against a resistance force. The lever amplifies either the magnitude of applied force or the range and speed of motion it produces. There are three types of levers:
- *First-class lever*: Axis is between applied force and resistance.

    Force amplification. When the axis is closer to resistance, the applied force has a longer lever arm; therefore, less force is required to overcome resistance.

    Motion amplification. When the axis is closer to applied force, resistance has a longer lever arm; therefore, greater force is required to overcome resistance, but the resistance moves through a larger range of motion or at greater speed than the applied force.
- *Second-class lever*: Resistance is between axis and applied force.

    Force amplification. Applied force has a longer lever arm; therefore, less force is required to overcome resistance.
- *Third-class lever*: Applied force is between axis and resistance.

    Motion amplification. Resistance has a longer lever arm; therefore, greater force is required to overcome resistance, but the resistance moves through a larger range of motion or at greater speed than the applied force.

Levers in the musculoskeletal system

Levers are commonly found in the musculoskeletal system: bones represent rigid bars, joints represent axes, and the external loads represent applied force, e.g. muscle contraction, and resistance, e.g. body weight and external contact forces. Most of the anatomical levers are third-class; this arrangement promotes the musculoskeletal system to be designed for speed and range of motion at the expense of force.

---

* Square brackets show SI (International System) units of physical measurements or chemical symbols of elements and compounds.

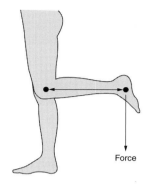

Fig. 1.6 Moment = Force × Distance

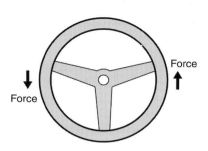

Fig. 1.7 A couple produces only a moment, but no resultant force, on an object.

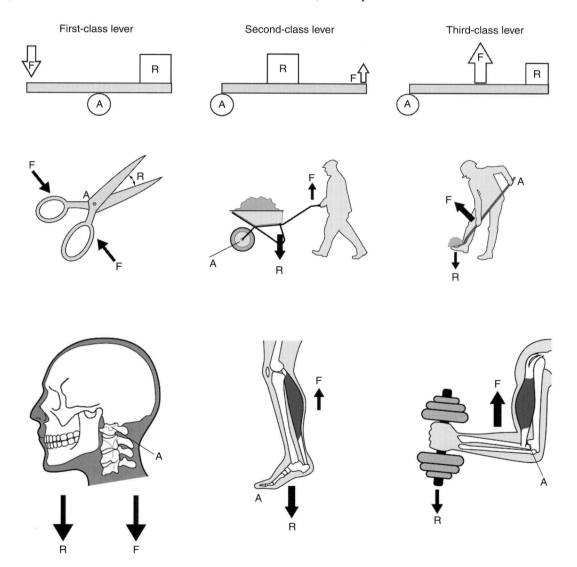

Fig. 1.8 A lever is a simple machine that operates on moments. The illustrations show the arrangement of axis (A), applied force (F) and resistance (R) in first-, second-, and third-class levers. Most of the levers in the musculoskeletal system are third-class.

Static analysis

Static analysis is an engineering method of analysing forces and moments produced when objects interact. There are a number of steps to applying static analysis.

Step one. A dynamic system is simplified to a static system at one instant in time. Therefore, all interacting objects are taken to maintain their relative positions.

This removes the need to deal with parameters of dynamic motion, such as displacement, velocity and acceleration.

Step two. As static analysis of all the forces in three dimensions is too complicated, the analysis is limited to the main (usually up to three) forces and their moments in one plane only.

In this step, the relevant 'co-planar' forces are isolated from the complex three-dimensional systems of forces.

Any 'simplifying assumptions' that have a bearing on the analysis are stated and their rationale explained, e.g. forces acting at an angle could be assumed to act in a vertical direction to make calculations manageable. A static situation can justifiably have different solutions, provided the supporting assumptions are valid.

Step three. A 'free-body force diagram' is drawn of the object under consideration, and all the forces acting on it are identified.

This is a simple but carefully drawn diagram, so that the forces are accurately represented in terms of their magnitude, direction and point of application with reference to the object. Newton's third law of motion is used to determine any 'reaction' forces acting on the object, e.g. ground reaction force.

Normally, more than one free-body diagram can be drawn for the same situation. The selection of free-body diagram for use often depends on the information available.

Step four. The conditions of equilibrium are applied to the free-body diagram, and any unknown forces and moments acting on the object are calculated.

Since the object maintains its relative position, the sum of all the forces and moments acting on it must be zero. This is the application of Newton's first law of motion.

The simplifying steps and assumptions applied mean that static analysis provides an estimation of the minimum magnitude of forces and moments acting on an object.

Free-body force diagram

A force is produced by interaction between two objects, and it acts upon one of them. It is ineffective to represent all the forces on all the interacting objects in a particular situation. Instead, a free-body force diagram is used to show all the forces acting on just one object. The free-body force diagram therefore isolates an object and the forces acting *on it* – this is an essential requirement before applying the conditions of equilibrium to the object.

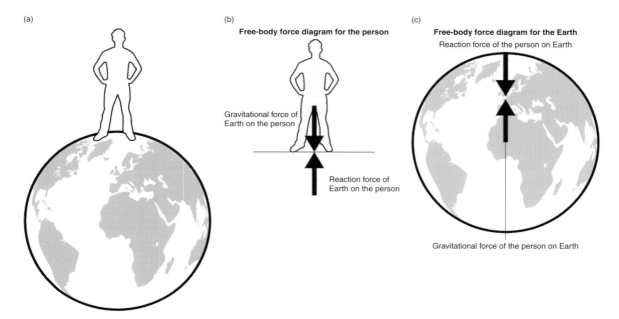

(a) (b) Free-body force diagram for the person (c) Free-body force diagram for the Earth

Reaction force of the person on Earth

Gravitational force of Earth on the person

Reaction force of Earth on the person

Gravitational force of the person on Earth

Fig. 1.9 A free-body force diagram is useful for isolating an object and the forces acting on it. It helps to simplify interactions between several objects. A simple example of a person standing on Earth involves four forces, which can be represented on separate free-body force diagrams for the (b) person and (c) Earth. It is first assumed that they are static with respect to each other, and that there are no other forces acting on them. Normally, only one of these free-body force diagrams is required, based on the object under consideration and information available.

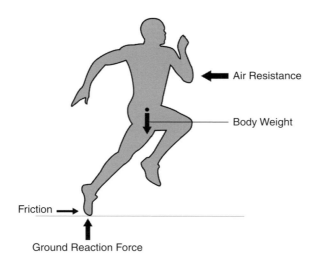

Air Resistance

Body Weight

Friction →

Ground Reaction Force

Fig. 1.10 This free-body force diagram shows the forces acting on a person whilst running. Here, a dynamic situation is simplified to a static situation at one instant in time. Although the force from air resistance acts over the whole body, in this free-body force diagram it is assumed to act collectively as a point load. In order to take a step forward, the person lifts one foot off the ground and pushes off with the other foot. The supporting foot exerts a contact force on the ground acting backwards. Friction is equal and opposite to this force and prevents the foot slipping backwards. Friction therefore acts forwards and provides motive force, i.e. a force that drives something forwards. The ground reaction force is equal and opposite to body weight. As this is a free-body force diagram of the person, it is not necessary to represent the forces acting on the ground.

Static analysis applied to the musculoskeletal system

Static analysis can be applied to the musculoskeletal system to estimate unknown forces, i.e. muscle and joint reaction forces, produced during normal everyday activities.

A number of simplifying assumptions have to be made in order to apply static analysis to a biological system in the same way as in general mechanics. The following general assumptions apply to most static analyses of the musculoskeletal system, and further specific assumptions must also be applied to each situation.

Static analysis

- The overall assumption in static analysis is that a limited two-dimensional analysis can provide a realistic estimation of the actual forces and moments.
- Average measurements of the human body, e.g. length and weight of limb segments, are usually taken from the reference anthropometric data.

Bones

- Bones are rigid bars of a lever. They transmit forces, but are not deformed by them.

Joints

- Joints are frictionless hinges. Other joint movements, e.g. rotation and translation, are ignored.

Forces

- Static analysis is commonly applied to the musculoskeletal system to estimate joint reaction force. Joint reaction force is an internal force in absolute terms, but is considered as an external force in static analysis. It is considered to be a compressive force that holds a joint together. All other internal forces are considered to cancel each other out (see page 5 for further information).
- The only external forces that can be applied to the musculoskeletal system are weight of the body segments, reaction force from other objects and muscle contraction.
- Muscles are the only soft tissues that actively produce force. Forces produced by other soft tissues, e.g. joint capsule and ligaments, are ignored.
- Muscles produce only tensile force, i.e. there is no compressive component to their action.
- The main group of muscles produces all of the force for a particular movement, e.g. triceps contraction produces elbow extension, and there is no other agonist or antagonist muscle action.
- The line of application of force is taken to be along the centre of the area of muscle cross-section. The point of application of force is where the muscle inserts onto the bone.
- All forces are taken to be as point loads, i.e. act at a specific point; instead of as distributive loads, i.e. act over a large area. The weight of an object or a body segment is taken to act at its centre of gravity. This is the average position of an object's weight distribution. In simple solid objects, e.g. a ball, the centre of gravity is located at the geometric centre; in objects with non-uniform weight distribution, it is closer to where most of the weight is located.

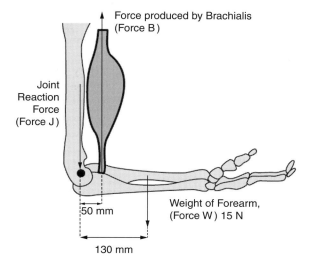

Fig. 1.11 Free-body force diagram of the upper limb showing forces acting about the elbow joint during flexion. The elbow is held at 90° of flexion. It is acting as an axis of a class III lever. The moment arm of the muscles is shorter than that of the weight of the forearm.

Assumptions

In addition to the general assumptions, the following specific assumptions are applied to this static analysis.

- Brachialis and biceps provide all of the flexion force.
- The force produced by brachialis and biceps is acting vertically upwards.
- The following physical measurements are based on anthropometric data:
  - Forearm mass is approximately 2.25% of total body mass. Therefore, in a 70 kg adult, forearm mass is assumed to be 1.5 kg. Assuming gravitational force is 10 N/kg, the weight of forearm equates to 15 N. This weight is assumed to act as a point load at the centre of the weight of the forearm, which is located 130 mm from the centre of rotation of the joint.
  - At 90° elbow flexion, the insertions of brachialis and biceps are 50 mm from the centre of rotation of the joint.

Calculations

Applying the conditions of equilibrium.

1. Sum of all moments is zero.
∴ Taking moments about the elbow joint:
Total clockwise moments = Total anticlockwise moments
$$15 \times 0.13 = \text{Force } B \times 0.05$$
$$\therefore \text{Force } B = 39 \text{ N}$$

2. Sum of all forces is zero.
$$\therefore \text{Force } B + (-\text{Force } J) + (-\text{Force } W) = 0$$
$$39 - \text{Force } J - 15 = 0$$
$$\therefore \text{Force } J = -24 \text{ N}$$

i.e. Force J has a magnitude of 24 N and is acting vertically downwards (hence the minus sign).

Elbow joint reaction force during flexion. This is an example of application of static analysis to the musculoskeletal system. It shows that the elbow joint reaction force is over one and a half times the weight of the forearm. This example also highlights the magnitude of loads acting on the joints of the musculoskeletal system. Most levers in the body are third-class, so most muscles have a shorter lever arm than the loads they are supporting. Therefore, in most joints, the reaction force is multiple times the weight of the supported body segments.

Simple machine

The concept of machine in mechanics

A machine converts energy from one form into another. Energy is the ability to do work. Work is done when a force moves an object:

$$\text{Work [J]} = \text{Force [N]} \times \text{Distance [m]}$$

Therefore, in mechanics a machine converts energy from one form into another by doing work, i.e. generating movement. This distinction is important because different types of machines convert energy from one form to another by different methods, e.g. a microphone converts sound energy into electrical energy.

Functions of a simple machine

A simple machine is a device that changes the magnitude or direction of a force. There are six classical simple machines, which are divided into two groups.

- Lever-based simple machines include lever, wheel and axle, and pulley. These simple machines use rotational movement to redirect a force.
- Incline plane-based simple machines include inclined plane, wedge and screw. These machines also redirect a force, but in a perpendicular direction to the original direction.

Simple machines can be combined together and with other devices to build more complex machines. In the most basic arrangement, a simple machine has two forces acting on it: an applied force that works against a resistance force. A simple machine is used to achieve mechanical advantage for work done by the applied force:

Work done by a force is the product of force and displacement of object:

$$\text{Work [J]} = \text{Force [N]} \times \text{Distance [m]}$$

Work done by both forces acting on a simple machine is the same, but a trade-off between force and distance is used to gain mechanical advantage for work done by the applied force. Therefore, a simple machine does not reduce the amount of work that is done, but changes the way in which it is done. Each simple machine has a specific mechanism, i.e. movement, that modifies the applied force.

As force and motion are connected, a simple machine can also be thought of as a device that modulates motion.

Sliding and rolling are examples of basic motions that displace an object. Simple machines can move an object by various means, e.g. a lever can produce rotational motion and a pulley can produce a lifting motion, and a screw can convert a rotational motion into linear motion. Simple machines, therefore, are the fabric of motion in complex machines.

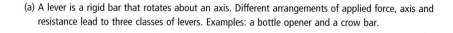

Simple machine

Mechanism of action

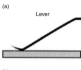

(a)

(a) A lever is a rigid bar that rotates about an axis. Different arrangements of applied force, axis and resistance lead to three classes of levers. Examples: a bottle opener and a crow bar.

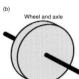

(b)

(b) The wheel and axle are a type of lever, as they also rotate about an axis. The axle passes through the centre of the wheel and both turn at the same time. Examples: a screwdriver and a steering wheel.

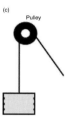

(c)

(c) A pulley is a variation of the wheel and axle. In a pulley, the wheel and/or the axle have grooves around the outside with a cord running through. A pulley can change the direction and/or magnitude of applied force. A 'pulley system' consists of two or more pulleys working together. Examples: a flagpole and blinds.

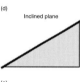

(d)

(d) An inclined plane is a flat surface that is higher at one end. It makes work easier by reducing the applied force needed to move a resistance. However, as in all simple machines, the smaller applied force has to travel a longer distance. In this case the applied force moves along the full length of inclined surface, whereas the resistance moves a shorter distance vertically. Examples: a ramp and a slide.

(e)

(e) A wedge consists of two inclined planes joined back to back. Therefore, a wedge is a type of inclined plane. It is used to do work by pushing the inclined plane into objects to split them apart. Examples: the blade of an axe/knife and a zip.

(f)

(f) A screw is really an inclined plane wrapped around a cylinder. The sharp edges of the inclined plane enable the screw to move in a linear direction as it is rotated. Examples: a light bulb and a jar lid.

Fig. 1.12 The six classical simple machines and their mechanisms of action.

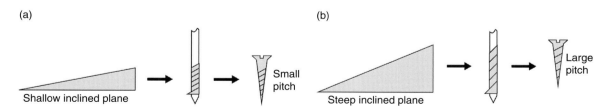

Fig. 1.13 A screw is an inclined plane wrapped around a cylinder.

Simple machines in the musculoskeletal system

The musculoskeletal system is a set of simple machines working together to support loads and produce movement. Only three types of simple machines are found in the musculoskeletal system: lever, wheel and axle, and pulley. These simple machines provide three functions:

- force amplification
- motion amplification
- change in the direction of applied force.

Most simple machines in the musculoskeletal system are designed to amplify motion rather than force.

Lever

Levers in the musculoskeletal system are discussed on pages 6–7.

Wheel and axle

This simple machine consists of two interconnected discs of different diameters with a common centre of rotation. Therefore, when either the wheel or axle turns, the other must turn as well, and both discs complete a turn at the same time. The wheel and axle are basically a form of lever, and their radii function as lever arms; usually, a wheel has a bigger radius than the axle. Force is applied to one component to overcome resistance acting at the other component. This arrangement provides mechanical benefits to the applied force as follows:

- *Force amplification.* Less force needs to be applied to the wheel to overcome resistance at the axle.
- *Motion amplification.* Greater force needs to be applied to the axle to overcome resistance at the wheel, but the wheel turns in a bigger arc at a faster speed than the axle.

In the musculoskeletal system, the wheel and axle arrangements provide amplification of both force and motion.

Pulley

A pulley is a device that supports the movement of a cord along its circumference. A force is applied to one end of the cord to overcome resistance acting at the other end. There is minimal friction between pulley and cord, and the cord transmits forces without stretching. A pulley produces mechanical benefits to the applied force as follows:

- A single pulley changes the course of the cord, and therefore the direction of the applied force.
- Multiple pulleys in series can change the direction and magnitude of the applied force: two pulleys in series halve the effort required to overcome the resistance, but the cord needs to move twice the distance. Similarly, as more pulleys are added in series, so the force required is divided, but the distance travelled by the cord is multiplied by the same number.

In the musculoskeletal system, a pulley is formed by bone, cartilage or ligament, with the cord formed by a muscle tendon. The tendon is lubricated to facilitate its gliding motion over the pulley.

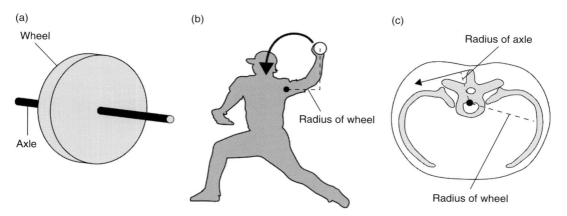

Fig. 1.14 Wheel and axle arrangements in the musculoskeletal system enhance range and speed of motion. The connection between the shoulder and the hand forms a wheel and axle arrangement: when the elbow is flexed to 90° degrees, the head of the humerus represents the axle, whereas the hand represents a segment of the wheel. A small turn of the head of the humerus produces a large corresponding movement of the hand, which increases the speed of action. Similarly, spinal muscles acting upon the vertebrae also operate in a wheel and axle arrangement: the spinal column represents the axle, whereas the ribcage represents the wheel. Small rotations of the vertebrae result in large corresponding movements of the ribcage. On the other hand, the action of oblique abdominal muscles attached to the ribs balances large forces produced by spinal muscles.

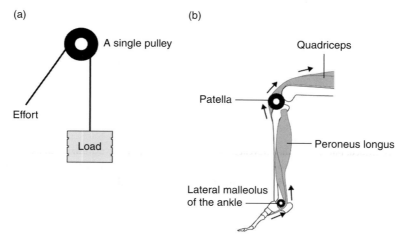

Fig. 1.15 Single pulley arrangements in the musculoskeletal system change the effective direction and efficiency of the applied force. The lateral malleolus and the peroneus longus tendon are an example of a single pulley arrangement: the peroneus longus tendon runs from the muscle on the lateral aspect of the leg, passes behind the lateral malleolus and inserts into the plantar aspect of the base of the first metatarsal. The muscle contraction therefore results in plantar flexion of the ankle and eversion of the foot. In the absence of the lateral malleolus, the tendon would have passed anterior to the ankle joint. The muscle contraction then would have produced dorsiflexion of the ankle and eversion of the foot. Similarly, the patella increases the angle of insertion of the patella tendon, thereby improving the direction and efficiency of the quadriceps force.

Stress and strain

The first section in this chapter explained that a force may have two effects on an object: it can change the shape and/or state of motion of the object. The previous sections were related to its effect on the motion of an object. This and the following sections relate to the effect of a force producing local shape change, i.e. deformation.

Force is a direct indicator of load in biomechanics. It is taken to act at a point when analysing its effect on motion of an object. However, it is usually integrated with other physical parameters to obtain derived measures of load when analysing its deforming effect.

Stress

Simply comparing two forces acting on two surfaces can be misleading because it does not take into account the size of the cross-sections. Stress relates the force to its area of application:

$$\text{Stress } [\text{Nm}^{-2} \text{ or Pa}] = \text{Force } [\text{N}] \text{ / Area } [\text{m}^2]$$

Stress indicates the intensity of force acting on a section. It is therefore a more fair comparison of loads acting on different surfaces. Although stress is derived from the applied force, it is actually a property of the object, i.e. stress is produced *within* an object by the applied force, and the same force can produce different stresses in different objects.

Strain

Strain is the deformation of an object due to stress. Strain is the ratio of change in length of an object to its original length:

$$\text{Strain} = \text{Change in length } [\text{m}] \text{ / Original length } [\text{m}]$$

Strain has no units. It is usually expressed as a ratio or percentage.

An object under stress experiences strain in the transverse direction as well as in the longitudinal direction. Transverse strain is usually opposite to longitudinal strain, i.e. as an object gets longer, it gets thinner and vice versa. Therefore, force can change the size of the cross-section it is acting upon. Still, stress and strain are usually based on the original dimensions of the object.

Although strain is a response of an object to internal stress, and therefore to the applied force, it can also be considered as a load in itself. This is further explained with the following example:

Adult cortical bone tolerates strains of only up to 2% before fracture. Conversely, strains at a fracture site must be less than 2% to allow cortical bone to form. This is due to the material properties of cortical bone, and is irrespective of its size. Therefore, a small bone, e.g. scaphoid, or a large bone, e.g. femur, would both tolerate strains of up to 2% before fracture. Therefore, biomechanical studies commonly consider strain (and strain rate) as an independent load, correlating it with other physical measurements, e.g. type of tissue formed at the fracture site, without directly going back to the stress or force producing the strain.

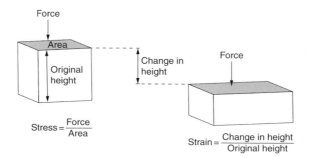

Fig. 1.16 The relationship between force, stress and strain. When considering the deforming effect of force, it is important to take into account the cross-sectional area over which the force is acting. Force produces stress along the entire length of the object, which leads to strain in the material. Note that the force changes the cross-sectional dimensions of the area it is acting upon.

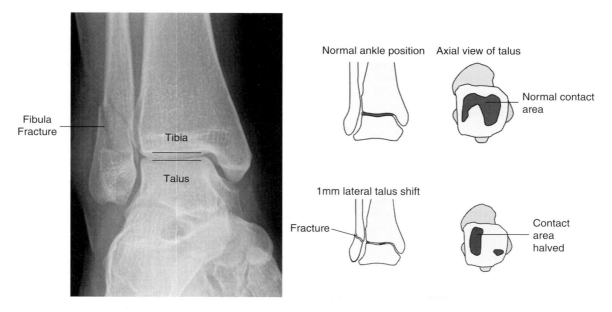

Fig. 1.17 Experimental studies have shown that an ankle fracture with lateral displacement of talus greatly increases the ankle joint load. In fact, a 1 mm lateral displacement of the talus can double the joint load in experimental models. In the normal position, the talar articulating surface is highly congruent with the tibial articulating surface, so the force on the talus is spread over a large area. A slight lateral displacement of the talus makes the articulation incongruent and dramatically reduces the talar contact area receiving the force, which doubles the stress acting on it.

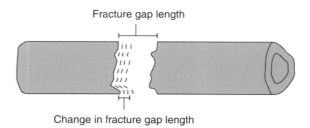

Fig. 1.18 Strain at a fracture site is described as the change in fracture gap length (due to motion of the fracture fragments) divided by the original fracture gap length.

Stress–strain curve

The stress–strain curve shows how a material subjected to an increasing tensile load deforms until failure. The calculations for stress and strain take into account the dimensions of the object, so the curve is characteristic of the material, and is not affected by the size and shape of an object.

The mechanical properties describe how a material deforms under load. The mechanical properties therefore determine the range of usefulness and service life of a material. The stress–strain curve describes a number of these mechanical properties:

- The initial linear section corresponds to elastic deformation. Strain is directly proportional to stress – this relationship is known as Hooke's law. The bonds between the molecules of the material are stretched but not broken.

  Therefore, deformation is temporary, and if stress is removed, strain is fully recovered and the material returns to its original shape and size.

  The gradient, i.e. steepness, of the straight line equates to the material's resistance to deformation. This is the stiffness of the material, and is technically described as 'Young's modulus' (or more correctly as 'Young's modulus of elasticity') or elastic modulus. The higher the Young's modulus of a material, the smaller the deformation produced for a given load.

- The yield point, or yield strength, is the maximum stress up to which a material undergoes elastic deformation. It is the limit of proportionality of Hooke's law, and beyond this point strain is not proportional to stress. Therefore, the material begins to 'yield' past this point.

- The non-linear section of the curve corresponds to plastic deformation. The molecular bonds are broken and the molecules move too far apart to return to their original positions. The deformation is permanent, and if the stress is removed, strain is not completely recovered and the material does not return to its original state.

  The ultimate tensile strength is the maximum stress that the material can sustain before fracture.

  The fracture point is where the material eventually fails. Stress at the fracture point can be slightly less than the ultimate tensile strength because the latter can cause the material to 'neck' (see pages 62–63), which reduces its cross-sectional area and therefore the force required to fracture.

- The area under the stress–strain curve represents the energy absorbed per unit volume of the material. It therefore indicates the energy absorbed by the material to failure. This is described as 'toughness'. A tough material takes a lot of energy to break it.

- Stiffness is an elastic property and strength and toughness are plastic properties of a material.

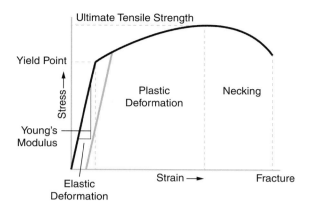

Fig. 1.19 The stress–strain curve defines the stiffness, strength and toughness of a material. These mechanical properties are determined by different sections of the curve: stiffness is defined by the gradient of the initial linear region, strength is the maximum stress that the material can withstand before failure and toughness is indicated by the total area under the curve. Different materials have different characteristics in these properties.

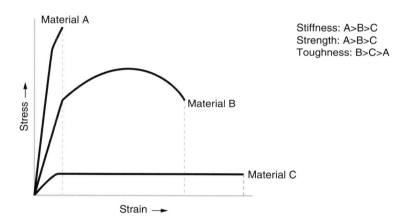

Fig. 1.20 Materials can be classified and compared with each other in terms of their mechanical properties. The stress–strain curves of three materials show that material A is the stiffest and strongest, material B is the toughest and material C is the most flexible (but weak). (Material A represents ceramics, material B represents metals and material C represents unreinforced polymers – these are discussed in the next chapter.)

Mechanical properties

The most commonly considered mechanical properties of a material are stiffness, strength, toughness, hardness and wear resistance. This section explains the connections and differences between them.

Stiffness vs strength

Stiffness and strength are often used interchangeably, but these are distinct mechanical properties. The commonest mistake is to refer to the strength of a material, when actually considering its stiffness. Stiffness is the material's resistance to change in shape and depends on elastic deformation. Strength is the load required to break a material and depends on plastic deformation. The stress–strain curve shows that a load that causes a material to fail must also take it beyond the yield point (i.e. its initial stiffness). For most applications, stiffness of a material is the more important mechanical property, i.e. a material must be *stiff* enough to not plastically deform under loads applied in its application. This is for two reasons, both of which relate to the stress–strain curve:

- The load range for elastic deformation is much greater than plastic deformation. Therefore, once a material passes beyond its yield strength, it is much closer to its failure point. It would be therefore unsafe to apply a material where it could yield, as a further small increase in load could cause it to fail. Therefore, in practical terms, the material's 'yield strength' is more important than its ultimate tensile strength.
- A material's behaviour is easier to predict in the elastic region, due to the linear relationship between load and deformation. Therefore, elastic deformation can be taken into account in the design of structures made from the material. However, it is more difficult to predict plastic deformation due to the non-linear relationship between load and deformation.

Hardness vs ductility

Hardness describes the material's resistance to localised surface plastic deformation, e.g. scratch or dent. Hardness is not a basic mechanical property, but instead is derived from a combination of other mechanical properties, e.g. stiffness and strength. Hardness determines the wear resistance of a material. Therefore, a harder material has a greater wear resistance than a softer material under the same loading conditions. Ductility describes the amount of deformation a material undergoes before fracture, e.g. a copper wire is very ductile.

Hardness and strength both measure plastic deformation of a material. Therefore, these are roughly proportional to each other, i.e. harder materials are generally also stronger. However, hardness and strength are gained at the expense of ductility, i.e. as the materials get harder and stronger, they generally become less ductile.

Toughness

Toughness is the material's ability to absorb energy up to the fracture. Toughness is derived from both strength and ductility of a material. Therefore, a tough material is normally both strong and ductile.

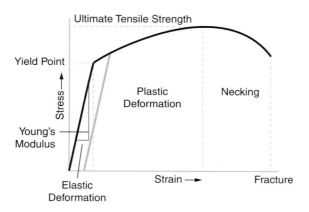

Fig. 1.21 Materials are generally only suitable for application under loads up to their yield strength. The elastic deformation range is therefore also known as the working range of a material. A material that is only elastically deformed returns to the original shape and size when unloaded. There is zero net work done over a loading cycle. The work done elastically deforming the material is stored as strain energy, which changes the material back to the original form when the load is removed. A material that is plastically deformed does not return to its original state when unloaded.

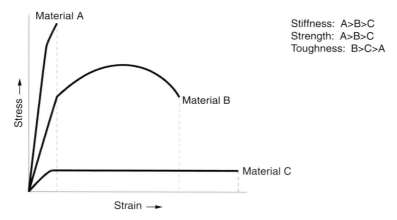

Fig. 1.22 Toughness is derived from both strength and ductility of a material. The stress–strain curves of three materials show that only material B is tough, Although materials A and C are both not tough, material A shows little plastic deformation whereas material C shows extensive plastic deformation. Material A is referred to as 'brittle' as it not very ductile. Material C is the most ductile of three materials, but it is not as tough as material B because it is not sufficiently stiff and strong.

Viscoelastic properties of materials

Mechanical properties describe how a material deforms under a load. Mechanical properties are not always constant, and may vary with external conditions, e.g. temperature. In other words, a material may show variable deformation behaviour under the same load, depending on the external conditions. In the same way, some materials also show variable deformation under the same load over a period of time or under different loading rates. Therefore, these materials display time-dependent, as well as load-dependent, deformation. Viscoelastic properties describe how a material deforms with time, and can be considered as extension of usual mechanical properties.

A material that displays time-dependent deformation is described as viscoelastic. Biological materials, e.g. bone, tendon and skin, are typically viscoelastic. Different materials have different mechanisms for their viscoelasticity.

Viscoelastic behaviour is commonly described in terms of four factors: creep, stress relaxation, strain-rate dependent mechanical properties and hysteresis.

Creep vs stress relaxation

If a viscoelastic material is placed under constant stress over a prolonged period, it shows increasing strain with time – this is creep. The technical definition of creep is that it is time-dependent deformation of a material under constant load that is below its yield strength. Therefore, creep produces plastic (i.e. irreversible) deformation of a material below its yield strength. Creep can eventually cause the material to fail. Therefore, creep can lead to failure of a material under loads significantly below its ultimate tensile strength.

Creep can be managed by reducing the applied stress over time. Stress relaxation is the decrease in stress required to maintain constant strain over time, i.e. prevent creep.

Strain-rate-dependent mechanical properties

The above section explained that strain in a viscoelastic material depends on not just stress, but instead is a product of stress–time combination. Time increases deformation produced by a given load. Therefore, a given load produces less deformation over a shorter time period than over a longer time period. Since stiffness is the resistance of a material to deformation, viscoelastic materials are stiffer when loaded over a short time period than over a longer time period. This demonstrates why many mechanical properties, e.g. stiffness and strength, of viscoelastic materials vary with the rate of loading. Typically, viscoelastic materials are stiffer, stronger and tougher when loaded at a faster rate, i.e. at a higher strain-rate, because there is less time for them to strain.

Hysteresis

Hysteresis occurs when a viscoelastic material is cyclically loaded and unloaded. It is the ability of the material to dissipate energy between the loading and unloading cycles. The dissipated energy is used to change the shape of the material during loading and unloading. As a result, further energy input is required to continue the loading and unloading cycles. Therefore, hysteresis allows viscoelastic materials to act as 'shock absorbers', e.g. intervertebral discs and menisci.

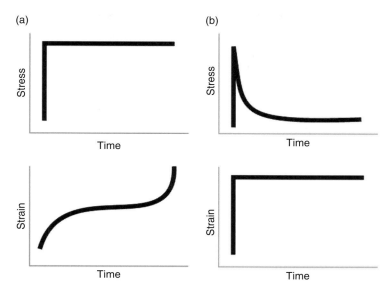

Fig. 1.23 These stress–time and strain–time graphs show the phenomena of creep and stress relaxation displayed by viscoelastic materials. (a) Creep is the time-dependent deformation of a material under constant stress that is below its yield strength. (b) Stress relaxation is the decrease in stress required to maintain constant strain over time, i.e. to prevent creep. Therefore, stress relaxation is the inverse of creep. A clinical example of application of creep response is the conservative treatment of clubfoot deformity in children. The plaster cast treatment applies constant load to lengthen the soft tissue over a period of time. The deformity is gradually corrected with sequential casting.

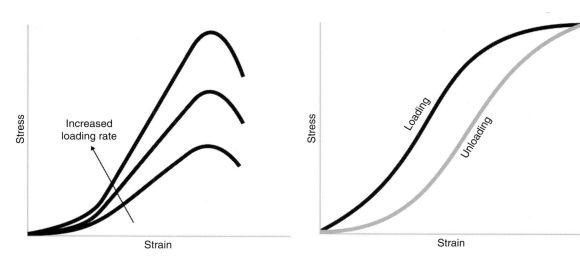

Fig. 1.24 The mechanical properties of viscoelastic materials vary with the rate of loading. Viscoelastic materials typically are stiffer, stronger and tougher when loaded at a faster rate, i.e. at a higher strain rate. Viscoelastic materials have both elastic and viscous properties; the viscous properties are influenced by the rate of loading.

Fig. 1.25 A viscoelastic material subjected to cyclical loading displays two stress–strain curves: a loading curve and an unloading curve, which form a 'hysteresis loop'. This is due to the fact that viscoelastic materials do not obey Hooke's law perfectly. The hysteresis loop shows that a viscoelastic material is harder to deform when loading than unloading. Hysteresis is the energy lost between the two cycles, and is represented by the area between the curves.

Structure and properties of materials

Our world is full of objects. These objects are made of different materials, which are composed of different internal microscopic structures. Therefore, all objects can be analysed in terms of their molecular arrangement. The properties and behaviour of materials is determined by the following structural factors:

- types of bonds between atoms, e.g. ionic or covalent
- arrangement of atoms, e.g. short molecules or long chains
- microstructure, e.g. crystalline or amorphous
- macrostructure, e.g. single crystal or polycrystalline.

This structural hierarchy divides all materials into four groups: metals, ceramics, polymers and composites. Materials in each group have similar molecular structure and therefore exhibit a similar range of properties. Material properties can be divided into chemical, physical, electrical and mechanical. These properties define how different groups of materials can be applied in the physical world.

A biomaterial is any substance, natural or engineered, that forms a part of either a biological structure or a biomechancial device that augments or replaces a natural function. All of the four groups of materials may be used as biomaterials. However, the properties of a material must be compatible with the body for it to be used as a biomaterial. Mechanical properties determine if a material can withstand applied loads and therefore define its practical functional capacity. Mechanical properties can be divided into two groups: static and viscoelastic (time-dependent). Static properties include stiffness, strength, ductility, toughness and hardness. Viscoelastic properties include fatigue, creep, stress relaxation and hysteresis. All these variables are just different measures of how the material deforms under load. This chapter looks into how the molecular structure of different groups of materials determines their mechanical properties and their applications in orthopaedics.

As well as being mechanically suitable, orthopaedic biomaterials should ideally also be biologically inert, easy to fabricate at reasonable costs and have appropriate handling properties. The biological environment can be highly corrosive, and orthopaedic biomaterials must also have high resistance against corrosion. All these requirements mean that the engineering materials that are practical for use in orthopaedic surgery are only a small fraction of the vast numbers that are potentially available.

An orthopaedic biomaterial must also be of 'medical grade', i.e. the type and quality of a material must meet a set of minimum requirements for medical use. In addition, stringent global manufacturing standards ensure that orthopaedic components are of high quality and have consistent mechanical properties and dimensional specifications.

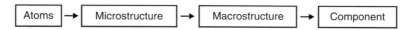

Fig. 2.1 All objects can be analysed in terms of their molecular arrangement.

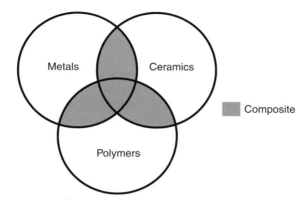

Fig. 2.2 A material is a physical substance used to make objects. There are four basic groups of materials: metals, ceramics, polymers and composites. Each group of materials has similar molecular and bulk properties.

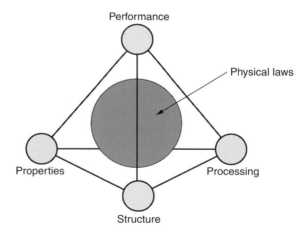

Fig. 2.3 This classical material science tetrahedron highlights that a material's structure, properties, processing (including application) and performance are all interrelated. Physical laws of biomechanics also have a bearing on these aspects.

Metals

Molecular structure

Metals typically have the simplest internal structural arrangement. They consist of atoms tightly packed together in a regular, repeating pattern to form a lattice. The lattices grow into crystals or grains, which are randomly and therefore evenly orientated in different directions. Metals therefore are polycrystalline materials.

The primary bonds in metals are metallic bonds: the adjacent atoms share an electron, and the whole structure consists of positive ions in a cloud of valence electrons. Metallic bonds characteristically are symmetrical, non-directional and moderately stiff and strong.

Metals initially appear to have a uniform, orderly structure. However, a large assembly of atoms inevitably develops imperfections. The different layers of atoms can become out of phase with each other and create defects within the lattice. In addition, the crystals also vary in size and shape. The junction between adjacent crystals is called a grain boundary. There is also misalignment between layers of atoms in different crystals at grain boundaries. All these imperfections affect the mechanical properties of metals.

Mechanical properties

Most metals have a higher density than non-metals due to the densely packed arrangement of their crystals. As a result, all metals, except mercury, are solids at room temperature. As there are numerous stiff primary bonds in a closely linked structure, metals as a group are stiff materials. The symmetrical and non-directional nature of primary bonds mean that metals have isotropic *elastic* properties, i.e. the elastic properties remain constant regardless of the loading direction.

Although metals as a group are stiff, strong and tough, pure metals are often too soft and weak for most practical applications. These *plastic* properties reflect the ease with which lattice defects move in pure metals when the primary bonds are broken. Most pure metals therefore require some form of 'treatment' to improve their strength, hardness and toughness to a useful level. A common method for achieving this is to transform pure metals into alloys.

The mechanical properties of metals (and other materials) change at elevated temperatures. This characteristic is used in the manufacturing process to prepare metals for fabrication work such as moulding, shaping and machining. The process of changing the mechanical properties of a material with heat treatment is called annealing. Annealing involves heating a material to above a critical temperature, maintaining that temperature for a set time and then cooling the material slowly. This makes the material softer and more workable.

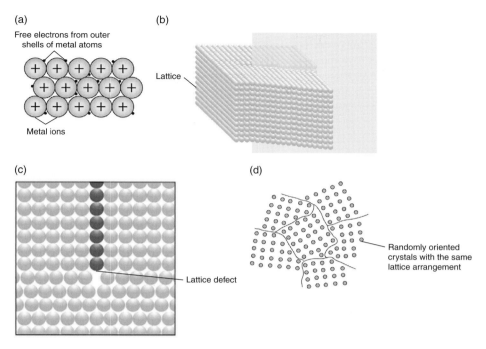

Fig. 2.4 Molecular structure of metals. Metals usually have atoms of (a) normally one element bonded together with metallic bonds, (b) into groups of lattices that (c) contain imperfections. (d) The lattices grow into crystals that are randomly orientated in different directions.

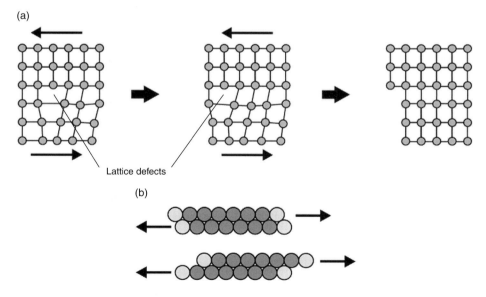

Fig. 2.5 Mechanism of plastic deformation in metals. (a) Plastic deformation in metals occurs when some of the primary bonds between the atoms are broken and the lattice defects are sequentially advanced until they reach the edges. (b) Otherwise, the movement of a whole plane of atoms over each other would require breakage of all primary bonds between the planes, which would require too much energy. (The three methods of strengthening metals discussed in the next section all involve restricting movement of lattice defects so that the yield stress (i.e. start of plastic deformation) is greater.)

Alloys

Highly pure metals are often too soft, weak, ductile and chemically reactive for practical use. Therefore, they are commonly mixed into alloys that have enhanced mechanical properties compared with the base metals. Alloys can be custom designed for a particular use more easily than sourcing a pure metal that meets the same requirements. Alloys can also be given specific properties during the development phase, e.g. resistance to corrosion. Therefore, almost all metals used in orthopaedics (and engineering) are alloys.

Molecular structure

An alloy is a substance that is composed of two or more elements, at least one of which is a metal, united by dissolving in each other when molten, e.g. brass is an alloy of zinc in copper. Therefore, an alloy is a 'solid solution' of different elements. The process of converting a pure metal into an alloy is known as 'solid–solution strengthening'.

The addition of a few 'impurity' atoms to a pure metal slightly distorts its internal structural arrangement. The host metal atoms still pack together tightly in lattices. However, depending on the size of the impurity atoms, these can replace or position themselves between the host atoms.

The primary bonds in an alloy are still the metallic bonds. An alloy also contains imperfections in the same way as a pure metal. However, the impurity atoms impose 'lattice strains' on the surrounding host atoms and impede the movement of lattice defects when the primary bonds are broken.

Mechanical properties

Plastic deformation in metals occurs by movement of lattice defects. The 'mis-fitting' impurity atoms impose restrictions to this process. Therefore, alloys are harder, stronger and tougher than pure metals. The fraction of impurity atoms can be adjusted to produce the most optimum combination of hardness, strength and toughness.

Other methods of strengthening metals

Pure metals (and alloys) can also be strengthened by two other methods.

Grain size reduction

Grain boundaries form natural barriers to the movement of lattice defects. Therefore, smaller crystals produce more grain boundaries that halt the movement of lattice defects. Smaller crystals are produced by a process called 'quenching', in which the metal is heated to above a critical temperature and then rapidly cooled down, so that there is less time available for the grains to grow.

Work hardening

This involves applying stress to a material until it plastically deforms and then removing the stress. Then, when the material is re-loaded, the deformation occurs at a higher yield point. Therefore, the material has effectively become stronger and harder. Plastic deformation works by increasing the overall number of lattice defects, thereby creating 'traffic jams' that obstruct movement of lattice defects.

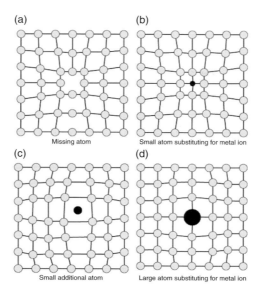

(a)   (b)

Missing atom   Small atom substituting for metal ion

(c)   (d)

Small additional atom   Large atom substituting for metal ion

Fig. 2.6 Mechanism of solid–solution strengthening. The impurity atoms in an alloy distort the lattice and significantly increase the resistance to movement of lattice defects. Possible mechanisms are shown above: (a) missing atom; (b) small atom substituting for a metal ion; (c) small additional atom; (d) large atom substituting for a metal ion.

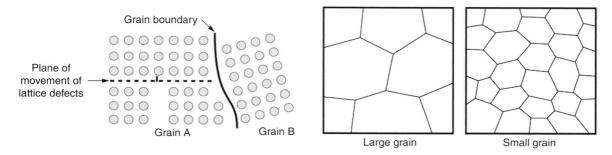

Fig. 2.7 and Fig 2.8 Mechanism of strengthening by grain size reduction. Grain boundaries act as natural boundaries to movement of lattice defects due to misalignment of atoms in different grains. Smaller crystals produce more grain boundaries, which make metals stronger.

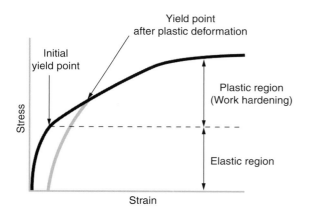

Fig. 2.9 and Fig. 2.10 Mechanism of strengthening by work hardening. A material that is plastically deformed and then unloaded has a higher yield point when it is loaded again. Strengthening by work hardening can be demonstrated using a wire or a paper clip. It is difficult to bend a straight portion back and forth repeatedly at the same place, because the strength of material increases with the work done. If this cycle is continued, the material eventually breaks due to fatigue failure.

Metals in orthopaedics

Three conventional alloys have obtained a wide use in orthopaedics: stainless steel, cobalt–chrome and titanium and its alloys.

Stainless steel

Stainless steel is used in making common surgical instruments and the temporary implants applied in trauma surgery, such as plates, nails, screws and wires. Stainless steel is easy to process, has good corrosion resistance in the biological environment and is relatively cheap. There are different grades of stainless steel and surgical devices are developed from the alloy type that has the most suitable combination of properties, e.g. surgical drill bits are made from stainless steel that is extremely hard and can be well sharpened (but it is also relatively brittle and the drill bits are prone to breakage without much deformation). The use of stainless steel alloys in developing long-term joint replacement prostheses has been limited because other alloys have better wear and corrosion resistance.

Cobalt–chrome

Cobalt–chrome alloys have the longest and broadest history of use in joint replacement prostheses. They are now mainly used to develop the metal-type bearing components of total hip replacements (i.e. the femoral head and acetabular cup). Cobalt–chrome alloys have very good wear resistance, fatigue strength and corrosion resistance. Therefore, these alloys are most suitable for making articulating interfaces of long-term joint replacement prostheses. However, they are not the best choice for making the stems of the prostheses. The stiffness of cobalt–chrome alloys is much greater than that of the cortical bone, which means that, if they are combined together, the prosthesis would take up most of the applied load. This would lead to stress shielding and resorption of surrounding bone, which in turn would lead to early prosthesis loosening.

Titanium and titanium alloys

Titanium and its alloys are comparatively new engineering materials that have an exceptional combination of properties. They are extremely strong, have half the stiffness of cobalt–chrome alloys and also have the ability to osteointegrate with bone. These properties mean that titanium-based implants can achieve good fixation with bone. Therefore, titanium alloys are the most appropriate materials for making stems of long-term joint replacement prostheses. They are also used to make implants for trauma surgery; however, these implants can sometimes be difficult to remove due to their osteointegration with bone. Titanium alloys have an oxide layer on the surface, which provides excellent resistance to corrosion.

The major limitations of titanium are its relatively poor wear resistance and high surface coefficient of friction. Titanium alloys therefore are not suitable for developing articulating components. Titanium-based implants are also prone to notch sensitivity, and any surface defects significantly increase the risk of fatigue failure. Titanium is also quite difficult to process during certain stages of manufacturing, e.g. forging and machining (Table 2.1).

Table 2.1. **Alloys in orthopaedics**

Alloy	Composition
Stainless steel	Steel is an iron–carbon alloy. Stainless steel is iron–carbon alloy that also contains chromium and sometimes nickel. It may also contain minor quantities of other elements, such as manganese, molybdenum and sulphur. Stainless steel has a high resistance to corrosion when compared with plain steel – this is a function of chromium and nickel. The different grades of stainless steel used in orthopaedics are broadly divided into two groups: • *Instrument stainless steel.* These alloys usually do not contain nickel. Therefore, their corrosion resistance is relatively low. These are extremely hard and can break relatively easily. • *Implant stainless steel.* These alloys contain nickel and therefore have greater corrosion resistance. These also have better fatigue strength and toughness. Newer stainless steel alloys containing high nitrogen content are being used in joint replacement prostheses. High nitrogen content makes stainless steel stronger and more resistant to localised corrosion than normal stainless steel.
Cobalt–chrome	Cobalt–chrome alloys consist principally of cobalt and chromium with trace quantities of other elements, such as molybdenum, tungsten and nickel. Cobalt–chrome alloys are very stiff and strong and are also used in gas turbines and dental implants. Their high corrosion resistance is a function of their bulk composition and surface oxide.
Titanium and Titanium alloys	Almost all of the commercially produced titanium is utilised in the aviation industry to produce high performance components for aircrafts and space vehicles. The quantity of titanium used in orthopaedics is a very small fraction ($\cong$2%) of the overall titanium usage. Therefore, titanium used in orthopaedics is of the same high standard as in the aviation industry. Titanium-based materials used in orthopaedics are commercially pure titanium* and its alloys contain small amounts of aluminium and vanadium. Titanium-based implants are comparatively very expensive because of the high manufacturing costs. However, these implants are compatible with modern MRI scanners, and can be used in patients with nickel allergy.

* It is not possible to obtain an absolutely pure metal, because these are extremely reactive and form an oxide layer.

Ceramics

Molecular structure

Ceramics are non-metallic materials produced with the use of heat, e.g. pottery made from clay. Common ceramics are compounds that consist of a metal combined with oxygen, carbon, nitrogen or sulphur, i.e. metal oxides, carbides, nitrides or sulphides, respectively. The combination of different elements means that ceramics are a large family of materials with varied and complex molecular structures.

The primary bonds in ceramics are ionic and/or covalent bonds. An ionic bond is formed by electrostatic force between positive (metal) and negative (non-metal) ions. Ionic bonds are symmetrical, non-directional and very stiff and strong. A covalent bond is formed when electrons are shared between non-metal atoms. Covalent bonds are variably spread (symmetrical/ unsymmetrical), very directional and very stiff and strong.

Ceramics can be crystalline, partially crystalline or amorphous. Crystalline materials consist of atoms arranged in regular lattices, e.g. NaCl. Amorphous materials have randomly packed molecules with no regularity in their spatial arrangement (amorphous means 'no structure'). Partially crystalline materials consist of a mixture of crystalline and amorphous phases.

Mechanical properties

Ceramics tend to be less dense than metals: ceramics with ionic bonds contain non-metals, which are generally lighter than metals; and ceramics with covalent bonds are less densely packed. Ceramics, like metals, have a network of primary bonds in a closely packed structure. However, ionic and covalent bonds are usually stiffer and stronger than metallic bonds. Therefore, ceramics are typically stiffer, stronger and harder than metals. They also have a greater resistance to wear. The strength of the primary bonds also means that ceramics have a high resistance to chemically reacting with other substances. Therefore, ceramics have excellent resistance to corrosion.

Ceramics are extremely brittle and do not deform significantly before breaking. This is because crystalline ceramics have a set structure that cannot be changed easily because rearrangement of positive and negative ions in a lattice or atoms joined through covalent bonds takes a considerable amount of energy, and amorphous ceramics do not have crystal lattices in which lattice defects can move. Therefore, ceramics have low fracture toughness and are highly susceptible to fracture.

In common with other brittle materials, ceramics are strong in compression, but weak in shear and tension. This is because ceramics contain impurities and defects (like all materials), which act to amplify stress and therefore reduce the overall strength (see pages 72–73 for further details on the effect of stress raisers). Stress amplification occurs mainly in shear and tension, but not in compression – compression, in fact, closes defects and reduces the overall number of imperfections in the material. Therefore, ceramics are about ten times as strong in compression as in tension (Table 2.2).

Table 2.2. **Basic chemistry**

A compound is a substance that is formed when two or more elements chemically react together to form an ionic or covalent bond. A compound usually has completely different properties from its base elements. The base elements in a compound cannot be separated by physical methods. This can only be done by further chemical reactions or by using electric current.

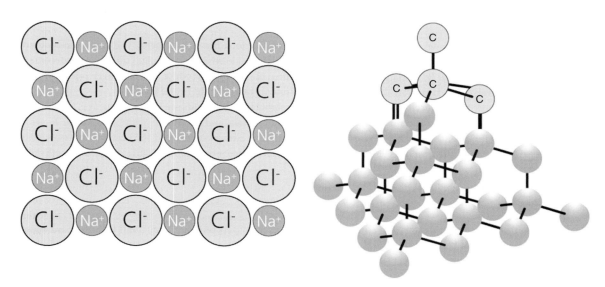

Fig. 2.11 Ceramics are earthly materials that consist of metallic and non-metallic elements. The primary bonds in ceramics can be ionic, as in sodium chloride, or covalent, as in diamond. Ceramics are characteristically hard and brittle materials.

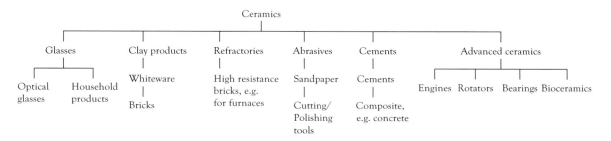

Fig. 2.12 Ceramics are a diverse group of materials. This chart shows the different classes of ceramics and examples of their uses in domestic, industrial and building products.

Ceramics in orthopaedics

Ceramics used in orthopaedics are classified as bioinert or bioactive. Bioinert ceramics show little or no chemical change in the biological environment and usually generate only a small, non-specific fibrous reaction in the local tissues. Bioactive ceramics chemically interact with the biological tissues. They are biodegradable and are slowly replaced by the natural tissues.

Bioinert ceramics

Bioinert ceramics are used for developing the bearing components of total hip replacement. The two main bioinert ceramics are alumina and zirconia. Alumina is used for both the femoral head and acetabular cup, whereas zirconia is used for only the femoral head. Both materials have a high degree of hardness, produce very low wear rates and have excellent corrosion resistance. However, they are also susceptible to catastrophic brittle fracture.

The lowest wear rates are produced when the femoral and acetabular components are both ceramic, i.e. in alumina-on-alumina combination. However, ceramics are much stiffer than metals, and in patients with osteoporotic bones, a ceramic acetabular component can produce stress-shielding and bone resorption around the acetabulum, which can lead to aseptic loosening of the implant. Therefore, a combination of zirconia head articulation with a polyethylene acetabular cup is also commonly used.

Bioactive ceramics

Bioactive ceramics have similar or identical composition to the mineral part of bone. They bond with the bone tissue and act as scaffold to stimulate new bone formation on their surfaces. Bioactive ceramics are osteoconductive, which means that they can only stimulate new bone formation within an osseous environment. In contrast, an osteoinductive substance (e.g. bone morphogenetic proteins) can stimulate new bone formation even outside the osseous environment. Bioactive ceramics are used as coatings on uncemented implants to enhance fixation and as bone substitute grafts to fill in bone defects until bone regenerates.

Ceramics used as bioactive coatings are calcium hydroxyapatite [$Ca_{10}(PO_4)_6OH_2$] and β-tricalcium phosphate [$Ca_3(PO_4)_2$]. They are applied onto implants in the form of a plasma spray to produce a 50–150 microns thick layer. They stimulate bone ingrowth and ongrowth to the implant surface, and therefore create a biological union between bone and prosthesis.

Bone substitute grafts are developed from calcium hydroxyapatite, β-tricalcium phosphate or bioactive glasses. Bioactive glasses are also ceramics and mainly consist of oxides of silicon, sodium, calcium and phosphate [e.g. $Na_2OCaOP_2O_3$-SiO], and gradually release these metal ions into bone. As ceramics are weak under tension and have low fracture toughness, bone substitute grafts are not suitable for load-bearing applications (Table 2.3).

Table 2.3. **Bioinert ceramics as joint-bearing surfaces**

Advantages	The wear of bearing surfaces of replacement joints is a big issue, as this leads to aseptic loosening of the prostheses. The main advantage of ceramics is that their very high hardness and low surface friction leads to much lower wear debris generation compared with other materials. However, although the mass of debris is low, the number of debris particles is high, i.e. the wear debris is very fine. Ceramics also have good biocompatibility and excellent corrosion resistance.
	Alumina = Aluminium oxide [Al_2O_3]. Naturally occurring alumina is better known as sapphire or ruby. Zirconia = Zirconium oxide [ZrO_2]. Alumina is harder than zirconia. Zirconia femoral head was introduced because zirconia has a superior wear resistance in a 'hard-on-soft' bearing combination. Therefore, zirconia-on-polyethylene combination produces far less wear debris than alumina-on-polyethylene combination. However, as zirconia has a lower hardness than alumina, it also has a lower wear resistance in a 'hard-on-hard' bearing combination. Zirconia-on-zirconia combination has a much higher wear rate than alumina-on-alumina combination, and therefore zirconia is not used to make the acetabular cup.
Disadvantages	As ceramics are brittle in nature, their main drawback is the risk of sudden and unpredictable fracture of the femoral head. It is important that, during the manufacturing process, ceramics have minimum impurities and defects introduced in order to minimise the impact on the ceramics' fracture strength. Therefore, ceramic bearing components are comparatively expensive to manufacture. 'Zirconia toughened alumina' composites have been found to have better fracture toughness than individual ceramics, and are also being used to produce the bearing surfaces. Modern ceramic femoral heads are individually tested to a load of about 25 times body weight before distribution to ensure that the risk of *in-vivo* failure is minimised. In 1998, when a manufacturer of zirconia femoral heads altered a single production step, it led to a surge in femoral head fractures (at least 343 reported cases worldwide). The company in question stopped making these implants. Studies show that the overall risk of *in-vivo* ceramic failure is in the order of 0.02%–0.7%.

Bioactive ceramics
Calcium hydroxyapatite is widely used as a bioactive coating for uncemented total joint replacements to avoid the problems associated with the use of cement. Calcium hydroxyapatite degrades on implantation approximately at the rate at which the new bone generates. Bone grafts are routinely required in spinal fusion, revision joint replacements, fracture repair and to fill bone defects, such as after resection of bone tumours. Currently, the source of bone for these applications is approximately 35% autografts, 60% allografts and 5% synthetic materials, i.e. bone substitute bioactive ceramics. Bone substitute grafts can be loaded with antibiotics or growth factors for local delivery at a controlled rate.

Polymers

Molecular structure

Polymers are large molecules that consist of long chains of repeating simple molecules (monomers). The process of monomers joining together to form long chains is called polymerisation. Copolymers are polymers made of two or more different types of monomers. Most polymers are organic and based on carbon atom monomers. As carbon atoms are usually also bound to hydrogen atoms, most polymers are hydrocarbons.

There are two types of bonds in polymers. Monomers forming the long chains are bound to each other by primary covalent bonds. Covalent bonds are stiff and strong and a chemical reaction is required to form or break them. The long chains stick together in groups due to secondary bonds formed by intermolecular attractions between molecules in adjacent chains. These secondary bonds (also known as van der Waal's bonds) are much less stiff and strong and can be overcome by mechanical methods. Primary covalent bonds may also link adjacent long chains to form a network of cross-links.

The long chains can have a variable structure. They can vary in length, degree of branching and the overall three-dimensional arrangement. The exact structure of chains depends on the conditions under which a polymer is synthesised. They can be randomly tangled to produce an amorphous structure or orderly arranged into a crystalline structure.

Polymers can be naturally occurring or synthetic. Naturally occurring polymers include proteins, DNA, rubber, wool and silk. Synthetic polymers produce a wide range of materials with many uses in everyday life, e.g. all plastics are polymers.

Mechanical properties

The mechanical properties of polymers depend on their molecular structure, loading mode and external factors such as time and temperature. In general, the structure of long chains affects mechanical properties of polymers as follows:

- *Length*. As chains become longer, polymers become stronger. This is because longer chains are usually more tangled, which allow more secondary bonds to form between chains.
- *Branching*. Linear, unbranched chains can pack more closely than branched chains; therefore linear chains produce crystalline polymers that are stronger.
- *Cross-linking*. As long chains become more extensively linked by primary covalent bonds, polymers become stiffer, harder and stronger.

As a group, polymers tend to be less dense than metals and ceramics. They are also not as stiff and strong as the other materials. However, they are extremely ductile and pliable and can be easily formed into complex structures. They have a low coefficient of friction and good resistance to corrosion.

Unlike metals and ceramics, polymers show viscoelastic behaviour, i.e. their stiffness varies with time. This is due to entanglement of the long chains, so that when the polymers are loaded, the long chains straighten out first before the secondary bonds are affected, which gives polymers variable stiffness.

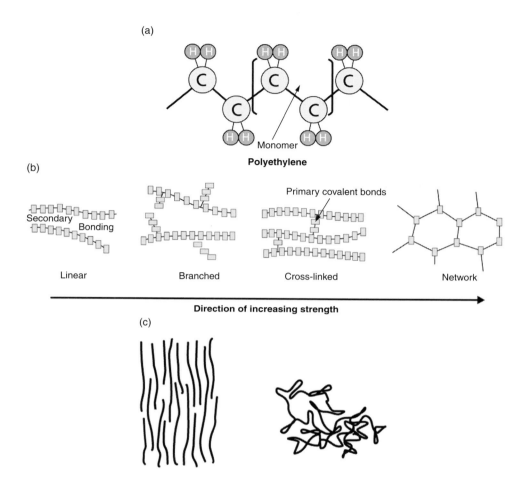

Fig. 2.13 Polymer = Many parts. A polymer is like a necklace made from small beads. (a) Polyethylene is the most common polymer, and consists of the ethylene monomer. Polymers are a large family of materials. Their mechanical properties depend on the nature of the monomer(s) forming (b) long chains and the number and type of bonds between the adjacent long chains. (c) The long chains can be packed together in an ordered or tangled fashion, producing a crystalline or an amorphous structure, respectively.

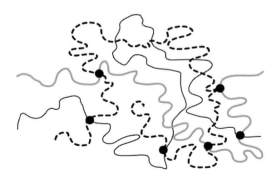

Fig. 2.14 Polymers show viscoelastic behaviour because of their tertiary structure. The long chains are loosely packed together in clusters. There are primary covalent bonds between monomer units forming long chains, and further bonds between chains, which can be the weak secondary bonds or strong primary bonds. When a load is applied, the polymer chains uncoil before the bonds break, which produces the viscoelastic behaviour.

Polymers in orthopaedics

Polymers used in orthopaedics are divided into two groups: long-term implantable and biodegradable polymers.

Long-term implantable polymers

Ultra-high molecular weight polyethylene (UHMWPE)

The main applications of UHMWPE are in the form of articular surfaces in joint replacements, e.g. acetabular component in total hip replacements, tibial insert and patellar components in total knee replacements and as a spacer in intervertebral disc replacements. It is suited to these roles because of its mechanical properties of good wear resistance and low friction. The main drawback of UHMWPE is the production of wear particles, which initiate an inflammatory response that, over time, leads to osteolysis and aseptic loosening of the prosthesis.

Highly cross-linked UHMWPE is an enhanced variety in which the polymer long chains are cross-linked extensively by primary covalent bonds. The long chains are therefore fixed in their relative positions and produce a greater wear resistance. Therefore, highly cross-linked UHMWPE is harder and has much lower wear rate than standard UHMWPE. However, the restriction in the movement of long chains also affects plastic deformation and makes highly cross-linked UHMWPE brittle.

Polymethylmethacrylate (PMMA) bone cement

PMMA bone cement is used to fix implants into bone in cemented total joint replacements. Although referred to as 'cement', it acts as a grout (space filler), rather than as an adhesive. It provides excellent primary fixation of the prostheses, but does not simulate secondary biological fixation. Therefore, the quality of fixation degrades over time.

PMMA bone cement comes in two parts: a powder phase and a liquid phase, in a ratio of 2:1 by weight. The main ingredients in the powder phase are:

- prepolymerised PMMA
- an initiator (benzoyl peroxide) to catalyse the polymerisation process
- +/− barium sulphate or zirconia to add radio-opacity
- +/− colouring agent, e.g. chlorophyll
- +/− antibiotics.

The main ingredients in the liquid phase are:

- monomer methylmethacrylate
- reaction accelerator (N-N-dimethyl-*p*-toluidine, DMPT).

The two phases are mixed together and a polymerisation reaction combines the monomer molecules to produce the final PMMA polymer. The ingredients initially form a paste – which is easily applied where required – and then harden and set by about 12 minutes from the start of mixing. The polymerisation reaction is exothermic and is associated with a sharp temperature rise.

Biodegradable polymers

Biodegradable polymers include polyglycolide (PGA), polylactide (PLA) and polydioxanone (PDS). These polymers have been developed into sutures, staples, pins, screws and plates. They provide temporary structural support and gradually undergo hydrolytic degradation. Biodegradable implants have several advantages over standard implants: they have less stress-shielding effect; they eliminate the need for surgical removal of the implant; and compared with metal implants, they have less interference with radiological investigations. The degradation times of devices are customised to titrate the load transmitted through the tissues and fixation device as the healing progresses (Table 2.4).

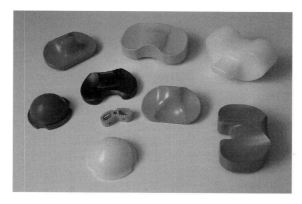

Fig. 2.15 UHMWPE consists of chains that are about 500 000 carbon atoms long. It is used to develop the bearing surfaces of total joint replacements. The newer highly cross-linked UHMWPE has much lower wear rates than standard UHMWPE, but is a more brittle and less forgiving material. (Photo reproduced courtesy of Cutting Tal Engineering/Bill Kennedy.)

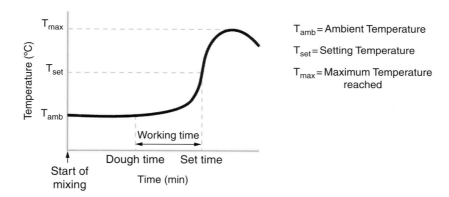

Fig. 2.16 The typical time–temperature curve for bone cement setting reaction. 'Dough time' is the time it takes for cement to reach a dough-like state. 'Set time' is the time it takes for cement to harden and set. 'Working time' is the interval between dough time and set time, during which cement can be applied and implants inserted and adjusted.

Table 2.4. **Bone cement**

Advantages	Flexibility of the procedure.
	Delivery of antibiotics to the site.
	Immediate stability of the components: patients can mobilise bearing full weight straight away.
	The use of cement is well established, and long-term outcome studies have been completed and cementing technique has been refined.
Disadvantages	Cement sets with a large exothermic reaction, which leads to local bone necrosis.
	Residual monomer can enter the blood supply, producing pulmonary embolism.
	Radiopacifier particles can reduce the mechanical properties of cement by up to 10% due to the discontinuities produced.
	Aseptic loosening in the long term.

Composites

Molecular structure

Composites consist of two or more base materials that remain discrete after they are combined together. The basic structure of a composite is that a 'reinforcement' material is dispersed in the volume of a 'matrix' material. The reinforcement material adds its mechanical properties to the matrix material, which supports the former by maintaining the relative arrangement of its fibres. When the composite is loaded, the matrix phase accepts the load over a large surface area and transfers it to the reinforcement phase.

There is usually no chemical bonding between the base materials. Instead, the matrix material 'melds' with the reinforcement material. This can occur in a number of ways, such as the matrix material simply solidifying from a molten state or there can be chemical polymerisation within the matrix material. This results in a mechanical bond between the two phases. However, there is still a clear interface between the two phases, and the materials can be readily distinguished if the composite is broken down.

The selection and composition of base materials depend on the composite's final desired characteristics. Composites are classified into three groups according to the type of material forming the matrix phase: metal matrix composites, ceramic matrix composites and polymer matrix composites. Most of the commonly used composites are polymer matrix composites. The two phases of a composite can belong to the same class of materials, e.g. a polymer can be the reinforcement phase within another polymer as a matrix phase.

Mechanical properties

Composites have enhanced properties compared with the base materials. This is based on the principle of combined action, so that the synergistic effect of the base materials produces better overall properties of the composite. Composites are considered in situations where the combination of required properties cannot be met by a single base material on its own. The biggest advantage of composites is that they can be stiff and strong but still very light, i.e. have high strength to weight ratio. Their main downside is the associated very high development costs.

The size and arrangement of reinforcement material have a huge influence on the properties of the composite. The reinforcement material can be in the form of particulates (filled composite), fibres (fibre composite) or continuous sheets (laminated composite). Composites usually have anisotropic mechanical properties that vary according to the orientation of the applied load to the alignment of reinforcement material. The interface between the base materials is particularly vulnerable under stress and composites are prone to failure by 'delamination' (i.e. separation) of the two layers.

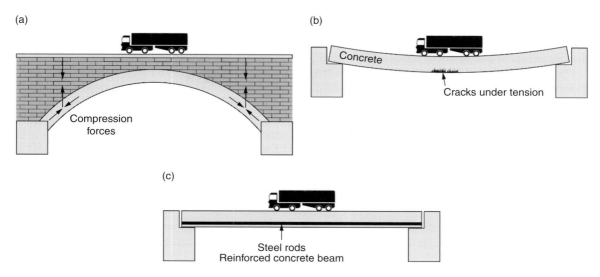

Fig. 2.17 Concrete is a composite of mainly crushed stones and cement. It is the most used synthetic material in the world. It is used extensively in the construction industry because it is cheaper than other materials and does not rust. Concrete is strong in compression but weak in tension. (a) An arch bridge is under mainly compressive loads, and therefore can be safely built from concrete. However, (b) a simple beam bridge is under compressive and tensile loads, and if built from concrete, its under-surface would crack and fail. (c) The solution is reinforced concrete, which is a composite of steel bars and plain concrete. Steel is strong in tension and supports the bridge at the tensile under-surface.

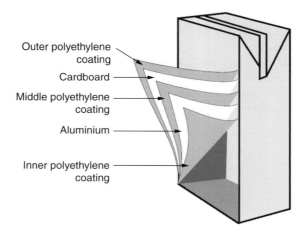

Fig. 2.18 A shelf-stable carton for storage of liquid contents is a laminated composite. It contains on average 74% cardboard, 22% polyethylene and 4% aluminium. The cardboard is a cheap, light and flexible material with adequate strength. The polyethylene coatings form waterproof barriers. The aluminium coating prevents oxygen diffusing through the container and causing the contents to oxidise and decay. Another example of laminated composite is plywood.

Composites in orthopaedics

Composites have a wide range of applications in orthopaedics. The following are a few examples of the more prominent uses of composites in orthopaedics.

Plaster of Paris is a composite of a fabric bandage (reinforcement phase) impregnated with gypsum cement (matrix phase). The gypsum cement forms a paste when mixed with water and hardens into a solid to form the required splints and casts. The newer synthetic cast materials are also composites that consist of fibreglass in a polymetric matrix.

Carbon fibre composites are gaining an increasing role in orthopaedics. They are already widely used in two types of orthopaedic hardware: in components of external fixators (pins, rings and bars) and in limb replacement devices (artificial limbs and braces). Carbon fibre composites typically consist of carbon fibres (reinforcement phase) in a polymer such as polyether sulphone (matrix phase). These composites have high stiffness and strength and low density. They also have excellent resistance to chemicals and heat, which is a function of the matrix phase. Together, this makes the devices produced lightweight, easy to handle, radiolucent and more durable. Lighter-weight devices reduce the energy expenditure during mobilisation. Therefore, limb replacement prostheses made from carbon fibre composites are better fitting and produce fewer sores and abrasions on limb foundation than the conventional heavier prostheses.

Carbon fibre composites also have an emerging role in the development of various other orthopaedic apparatus, such as in components of the operating table, instruments (e.g. screwdrivers, taps and drills), and in internal fixation implants (e.g. plates and nails). Carbon fibre equipments are lighter and radiolucent, and therefore are easy to handle and do not obstruct intra-operative fluoroscopic imaging. Implants made from carbon fibre composites have a stiffness similar to bone, and therefore are less likely to cause stress-shielding of bone or produce a fracture from a stress raiser effect. Carbon fibre fatigue resistance is also far superior to that of conventional materials. In addition, as the implants are radiolucent, the anatomical structures can be seen clearly, despite the intervening implants. However, radio-opaque marks are added to the implants to define their outline in radiographs.

Another application of composites in orthopaedics is in the form of synthetic sutures. As an example, FibreWire® is a suture that is a laminated composite of UHMWPE core covered in a braided jacket of polyester and UHMWPE. This combination of materials produces a suture with superior strength and abrasion resistance superior to conventional materials. It is used in situations where high strength repairs are required.

Finally, a composite is also formed when an implant, such as a plate, nail or prosthesis, is applied to bone. This is a laminated composite where the two materials are arranged in distinct layers. The bone–implant composite has different mechanical properties to the individual components (Tables 2.5, 2.6).

Table 2.5. **Plaster of Paris**

The chemical name of plaster of Paris is calcium sulphate; it is commercially also known as gypsum plaster. The term plaster of Paris comes from Paris, France, where it was first widely used in construction, art and medicine. However, it has been in medical use since 1852, when Mathysen, a Dutch military surgeon, used plaster of Paris bandages to make splints. The plaster of Paris bandage consists of a roll of muslin stiffened by dextrose or starch (reinforcement phase) and impregnated with gypsum cement (matrix phase). The gypsum applied to the bandages is anhydrous (dry) and produced by heating crystalline gypsum to around 150°C:

$$2CaSO_4 \cdot 2H_2O + Heat \rightarrow 2CaSO_4 \cdot \frac{1}{2}H_2O + 3H_2O$$

(**Crystalline gypsum**) (**Anhydrous gypsum**)

This reaction is reversed when water is added back to anhydrous gypsum. The average setting time for plaster of Paris is between 3 and 9 minutes. Movement of the material whilst it is setting grossly weakens the cast. The setting time is increased with the use of cold water or addition of sugar into water, and is reduced with the use of hot water or addition of salt into water. The average drying time for plaster of Paris is between 24 and 72 hours. The cast achieves its optimal strength when it is completely dry.

Table 2.6. **Fibre-reinforced polymer composites**

Glass fibre-reinforced polymer (GFRP). This is popularly known as fibreglass, and is one of the commonest composites. It consists of glass fibres embedded in a polymeric matrix. Glass fibres are stiff, strong and brittle, whereas the polymer is flexible, weak and ductile. GFRP has a combination of these properties.

Carbon fibre-reinforced polymer (CFRP). This consists of carbon fibres embedded in a polymeric matrix. CFRP is stiffer and stronger than GFRP. CFRP in fact has one of the best strength to weight ratio of all engineering materials. It is also used in the aerospace industry and in advanced sporting equipment. The main drawbacks of CFRP are that it is relatively brittle and much more expensive to produce than GFRP.

Bone I

Molecular structure

Bone is a highly specialised connective tissue. It is a biological composite, and its structural arrangement is much more complex than that of the engineering composites. Like all connective tissues, it consists of cells and an organic extracellular matrix. However, in addition uniquely it also has a high content of inorganic mineral salts.

In terms of a composite, bone consists of mineral salts (ceramics) as the reinforcement phase and collagen proteins (polymers) as the matrix phase. The mineral salts take the form of small crystals and are arranged in an orderly pattern within a collagen protein network. The key mineral salts present in the bone are calcium phosphate (hydroxyapatite) and calcium carbonate, and the collagen proteins are organised into type 1 collagen fibres. The mineral salts contribute stiffness and hardness to the strength and toughness of collagen fibres. The hydroxyapatite-reinforced collagen fibres form the basic 'building block' of bone.

At the microscopic level, bone has the structure of a laminated composite, which provides it with an extraordinary resistance to fatigue failure. The reinforced collagen fibres are organised into separate layers (laminae) of sheets and cylinders (osteons with central Haversian canals), which must all be individually broken to completely fracture the bone. As a result, although bone is filled with microscopic defects, its laminated organisation prevents bones from progressing into complete fractures under normal conditions.

At the macroscopic level, bone consists of two distinct types of tissues: cortical (compact) bone and cancellous (trabecular) bone. These are also organised into separate layers, which enhances the bone's laminated structure. Cortical bone forms the walls of the bone. It is dense (5%–30% porous) and stiff and is similar to very hard plastic. Cancellous bone occupies the central space within the bone. It is much less dense (90% porous) but considerably more malleable. The mechanical properties of the two tissues are determined by their density.

Bone is a dynamic tissue and its base materials are in a state of constant turnover. The osteoclasts dissolve the minerals and collagen, and the osteoblasts lay down new minerals and collagen. This remodelling process enables the bone to alter its configuration (composition and/or shape) in response to the functional demands. This connection between bone remodelling and the applied load is summarised by Wolff's law, which states that the rate of bone turnover is proportional to the mechanical stresses experienced by the bone. Therefore, bone adapts to produce the minimum-mass structure to withstand any sustained applied load.

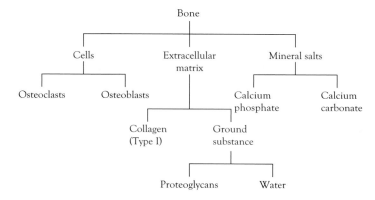

Fig. 2.19 The composition of bone. Bone consists of approximately 45% mineral salts, 35% collagen proteins and 20% water by weight.

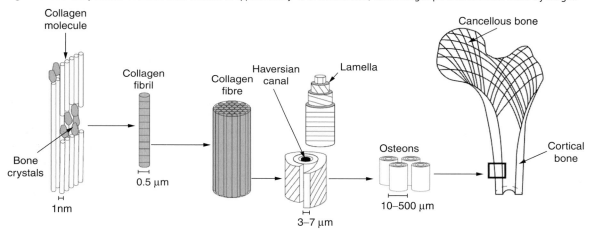

Fig. 2.20 The hierarchical structural organisation of bone gives it exceptional characteristics. It is very light for a structure that has the mechanical properties equivalent to that of reinforced concrete. In fact, the entire human skeleton makes up only about 20% of the total body mass.

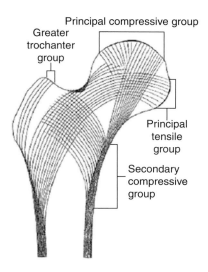

Fig. 2.21 The trabecular patterns in the proximal femur are the result of bone remodelling according to the loads sustained. Wolff's law explains the variation in bone density in different regions of the same bone, and the changes in bone density after prolonged periods of disuse or increased use.

Bone II

Mechanical properties

Bone is the third hardest structure in the body, after only dentine and enamel found in the teeth. However, the most essential mechanical property of bone for its daily functions is the stiffness. The stiffness of bone enables it to resist deformation under load and maintain the body's upright posture. The composite arrangement of different materials gives bone its complex and versatile mechanical properties.

In common with most engineering materials, stiffness and brittleness of bone are interrelated, which in the case of bone are a measure of its ceramic mineral contents. The dramatic effects produced by the change in mineral contents on bone's overall properties are observed between immature and mature bone. In children, immature bone consists mostly of collagen and is relatively less mineralised, but in adults mature bone has the opposite composition. As a result, immature bone is much less stiff but pliable, whereas mature bone is very stiff but brittle. These are optimum mechanical properties for the two different types of functional demands: children are involved in frequent, low-energy injuries, whereas adults need more support, speed and agility. The other important mechanical characteristic that bone inherits from its mineral contents is its variable strength: just like ceramics, bone is strong in compression but weak in tension and shear.

Bone is also anisotropic and viscoelastic. These properties are derived mainly from its collagen composition. Reinforced collagen fibres are aligned longitudinally. These fibres are essentially long chains of polymers. There are primary covalent bonds between the molecules of the chains, but mainly secondary bonds between adjacent chains. Therefore, a longitudinally applied load is working against stiff and strong bonds, whereas a transversely applied load is working against much weaker bonds. Bone is therefore stiffer when loaded longitudinally than transversely (anisotropy).

Polymers are characteristically viscoelastic due to their molecular arrangement. Polymers have complex tertiary structures so that long chains are loosely tangled together. When a load is applied, these chains uncoil before secondary and then primary bonds are broken. A longer period of loading allows the chains to unravel further, producing more deformation than a shorter period of loading. It follows that collagen fibres and therefore bones become stiffer, stronger and tougher at higher rates of loading (viscoelasticity).

The mechanical properties of bone change due to degenerative changes in the ageing bone. The cortical and cancellous sections are less dense in the ageing bone; therefore ageing bone becomes weaker, less stiff and more brittle.

For all of the above reasons, there is no single value for stiffness, strength and hardness of bone.

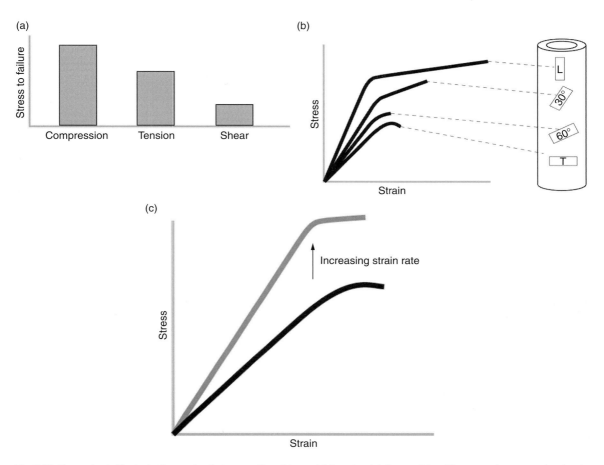

Fig. 2.22 These charts illustrate the mechanical properties of bone. (a) Bone is a brittle material and is stronger in compression than in other loading modes. (b) It is stiffer and stronger when loaded longitudinally than transversely (anisotropy) and (c) at higher rates of loading (viscoelasticity). (L = Longitudinal stress; T = Transverse stress)

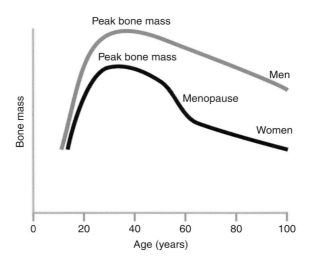

Fig. 2.23 Bone mass life cycle. The mechanical properties of bone are a function of its mass and therefore density. Stiffness and strength of bone vary with the third power and square of its density, respectively.

Further reading

Ann KN, Hui FC, Murrey BF *et al.* (1981). Muscles across the elbow joint: a biomechanical analysis. *J Biomech.* **14**: 659–696.

Bucholz RW, Heckman JD, Court-Brown CM (eds) (2006). *Rockwood and Green's Fractures in Adults.* 6th edn. Philadelphia: Lippincott, Williams and Wilkins.

Callister, WD (2007). *Material Science and Engineering: An Introduction.* 7th edn. New York: Wiley.

Curry JD (2006). *Bones: Structure and Mechanics.* London: Princeton University Press.

Dobson K, Grace D, Lovett DR (1998). *Collins Advanced Science – Physics.* London: Collins.

Floyd RT, Thompson CW (2011). *Manual of Structural Kinesiology.* 18th edn. London: McGraw-Hill.

Golish SR, Mihalko WM (2011). Principles of biomechanics and biomaterials in orthopaedic surgery. *JBJS-A.* **93**(2): 207–212.

Hall, SJ (1999). *Basic Biomechanics.* 3rd edn. London: McGraw-Hill.

Johnson K (2001). *Physics for You.* London: Nelson Thornes.

Johnson K (2006). *New Physics for You.* London: Nelson Thornes.

Johnson K, Hewett S, Holt S, Miller J (2000). *Advanced Physics for You.* London: Nelson Thornes.

Kutz M (2002). *Standard Handbook of Biomedical Engineering and Design.* New York: McGraw-Hill.

McLester J, Pierre PS (2008). *Applied Biomechanics: Concepts and Connections.* New York: Thomson Wadsworth.

Miles AW, Gheduzzi S (2012). Basic biomechanics and biomaterials. *Surgery.* **30**(2): 86–91.

Navarro M, Michiardi A, Castano O, Planell JA (2008). Biomaterials in orthopaedics. *J R Soc Interface.* **5**(27): 1137–1158.

Nordin M, Frankel VH (2001). *Basic Biomechanics of the Musculoskeletal System.* 3rd edn. London: Lippincott, Williams and Wilkins.

Ramachandran M (ed) (2007). *Basic Orthopaedic Sciences: The Stanmore Guide.* London: Hodder Arnold.

Rodriguez-Gonzalez FA (2009). *Biomaterials in Orthopaedic Surgery.* New York: ASM International.

Watkins J (1999). *Structure and Function of the Musculoskeletal System.* New York: Human Kinetics.

Mechanical properties of common orthopaedic biomaterials

Material	Elastic modulus (GPa)	Yield strength (MPa)	Ultimate tensile strength (MPa)
Alumina (Purity level 99.5%)	394	–	260–300
Bone cement (Polymethylmethacrylate)	3.5	20	70
Cobalt–Chrome (F75*)	220–230	275–1585	600–1785
Cancellous bone	1–11	–	2–20
Cartilage	0.02	–	4
Cortical bone	7–30	80	50–100
Plaster of Paris	1	20	70
Polyethylene	1	20	40
Stainless steel (316L*)	205–210	170–750	465–950
Titanium (Grade 4*)	105	692	785
Titanium (Ti-4Al-6V*)	110	850–900	960–970
Zirconia	207	–	248

Notes:

The values provided are for comparison only; the actual properties of any material depend on a number of factors, e.g. composition of constituents and processing conditions.

* This is the composition of alloy most widely used in orthopaedics.

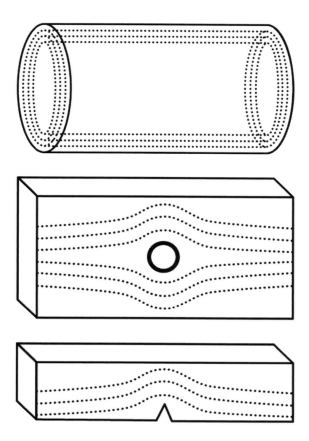

This diagram highlights that physical structures are non-uniformly loaded. Bending and torsional loads produce most of the stress on the surface of a structure. So, a hollow tube, such as a long bone, can be almost as stiff and strong as a solid tube of similar size, but being composed of less material is lighter. Also, structures naturally contain geometric flaws, such as voids and notches, which can cause local concentration of stress to several times the average stress level in the material, e.g. a hole can concentrate stress by a factor of three. These factors influence the design, application and performance of orthopaedic devices.

Introduction

This chapter develops on from the force–material interactions considered in the previous chapters. It looks into how solid structures withstand various types of forces. There are four basic modes of loading: compression, tension, bending and torsion. One mode usually dominates in a given loading situation. Therefore, structures can be labelled to highlight their loading mode:

- Columns carry compressive forces.
- Ties carry tensile forces.
- Beams carry bending forces.
- Shafts carry torsional forces.

The applied forces generate stress within the structure. The performance of a structure then depends on the properties of the material that it is made from, i.e. material properties, and how and where that material is distributed, i.e. geometric properties.

Material properties

Material properties determine the overall characteristics or personality of a structure. Material properties are the mechanical properties derived from the stress–strain curve, e.g. stiffness, strength and toughness. These properties determine how a structure performs under different types of load, e.g. ductile materials withstand tension better than brittle materials. Material properties are intrinsic to each material and are unaffected by how the material is used. The structure fails when the stress produced within the material reaches its failure limit. Therefore, material properties set the stress limit at which a structure fails. These properties have been considered in detail in the previous chapters.

Geometric properties

The size and shape of a structure determines how much stress (and strain) is produced in the material under a given force. The orientation of the applied force to the structure also affects the internal stress levels. The geometric properties therefore manage the stress levels in a structure.

Geometric properties can be considered in relation to cross-sectional and longitudinal profiles. Both profiles have a significant bearing on the load-carrying capacity of a structure. However, cross-sectional geometry has a more direct interaction with the applied force, because the cross-section of a structure forms the plane to which the load is applied, i.e. the plane of loading. Therefore, cross-sectional geometry is further considered in the analyses of the mechanics of different modes of loading. It is assumed that the cross-sectional geometry remains constant along the entire length of a structure.

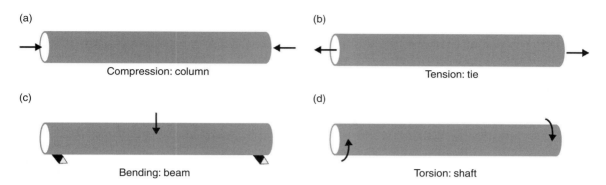

Fig. 3.1 There are four basic modes of loading. Structures can be labelled to highlight their function.

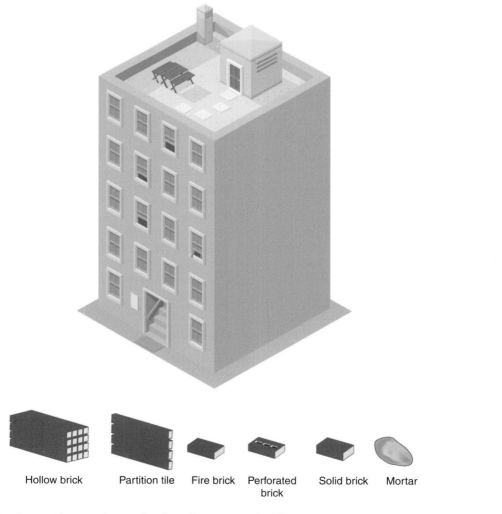

Fig. 3.2 Material and geometric properties together determine a structure's ability to carry loads. It is similar to how the physical properties of a building are a product of the properties of the building materials and the properties of the completed structure.

Compression and tension

Solid structures that carry compressive forces are referred to as columns, and those that carry tensile forces are referred to as ties. When considering the deforming effects of a force, it is important to define the alignment of the force to the structure.

Axial vs transverse force

An axial force acts along the axis of the structure. A transverse force acts perpendicular to the axis of the structure.

Normal vs shear force

A normal force acts perpendicular to the plane of loading. Stress produced by a normal force is termed 'direct' stress. A shear force acts parallel to the plane of loading. A shear force produces shear stress. Direct stress changes the shape and volume of a structure, whereas shear stress only changes the shape.

Compression vs tension

A compressive force is directed towards the centre of a structure and acts to flatten or squeeze it. A tensile force is directed away from the centre of the structure and acts to pull it apart. Compression and tension by arrangement are axial and normal forces. Similarly, compressive and tensile stresses are normal stresses. On the other hand, a transverse force by arrangement is a shear force and produces shear stress.

Stresses produced by compression and tension

Both types of forces generate stresses within the structure. Just as orientation of applied force to the plane of loading affects whether the force and stress produced are normal or shear, changing the orientation of a plane within the structure to the applied force also affects the type of force and stress acting on that phase. Therefore, different planes within a structure experience different combinations of forces and stresses.

These physical principles are put together to derive the following fact about compressive and tensile loading: under normal tension or compression, the plane of maximum shear stress is at 45° to the axis of loading. This is because a force as a vector quantity can be broken down into its component forces. The magnitude of a component force is highest at 45° to the applied force. Therefore, the plane at 45° to the applied force experiences maximum shear stress. Mathematically, maximum shear stress is always exactly half the normal stress. However, physical structures resist shear least well and often fail along the plane of maximum shear stress.

The effect of cross-sectional geometry on the properties of a column or tie

The strength of a structure under tension or compression is proportional to its cross-sectional area. Stress is calculated by dividing force over area; therefore the larger the cross-sectional area, the less the stress produced under a given force. A solid column is thus stronger than a hollow column of a similar size; it has more area and mass to withstand the applied force.

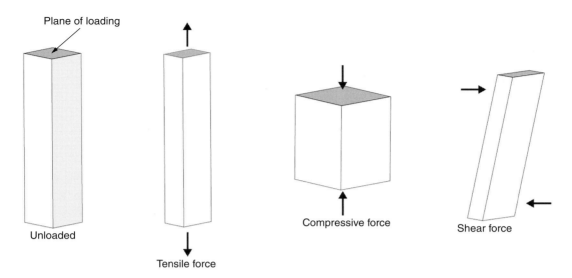

Fig. 3.3 The alignment of force to the structure is important when considering the deforming effect of the force. An axial force acts along the axis of the structure, whereas a transverse force acts perpendicular to the axis of the structure. A normal force acts perpendicular to a plane of loading, whereas a shear force acts parallel to it. An oblique plane within a structure experiences a combination of normal and shear forces and stresses.

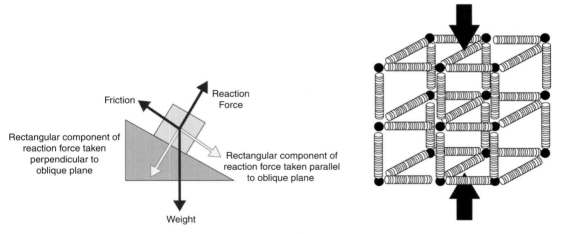

Fig. 3.4 A free-body force diagram of an object on an inclined surface. Reaction force from the surface on the object is a normal force, whereas friction is a shear force. Weight always acts in a vertical direction. It can be divided into its rectangular components, which here are taken to be perpendicular and parallel to the inclined surface. The perpendicular component of weight is equal and opposite to the reaction force. The parallel component of force is equal and opposite to friction. All forces are balanced and the object is in equilibrium. This example shows that a plane that is at an oblique angle to a force, in this case the inclined plane in relation to weight, is subjected to a combination of normal and shear component forces of that force.

Fig. 3.5 This basic spring-ball model roughly shows how an applied force produces different types of stresses along different planes within a structure. Here, the applied force produces compression, tension and shear stresses in springs in different planes. The structure would fail along the plane of springs that resists the internally generated stresses least well; this is not necessarily the plane of the applied force. Compression, tension and shear are the basic stresses, i.e. deformation mechanisms. Other loading modes act through a combination of these stresses.

Bending I

A beam is a solid structure that supports bending forces. The beam's length is considerably longer than its cross-sectional dimensions; typically at least ten times longer.

Beams are classified according to how they are supported. The basic types are as follows:

- *Simple (or simply supported) beam:* This spans two simple supports.
- *Cantilever beam:* This has a fixed support at one end and no support at the other end.
- *Overhanging beam:* This spans two simple supports with one or both ends extending beyond the supports.

Mechanics of a beam

This section describes the internal and external forces acting on a beam. A beam works by transferring the applied bending force as a compression force to adjacent supports. The applied force is transverse and acts perpendicular to the axis of the beam. It is therefore a shear force. It produces two types of internal forces within the beam: shear forces and bending moments. These internal forces are then transferred to the supports. Then, according to Newton's third law, the supports also exert an external reaction force back to the beam. Therefore, a beam is subjected to two types of external forces: applied and reaction forces. When combined together, the reaction forces are equal and opposite to the applied forces, and therefore the beam is in equilibrium.

The internal forces are not uniformly distributed, but instead vary along the length of the beam. These are usually represented in shear force and bending moments' diagrams.

Simple beam theory

Simple beam theory describes the stresses produced by bending forces. A simple beam with a single applied force is subjected to three points of loading (also known as three-point bending). The applied force produces compressive stress on its side and tensile stress on the opposite side of the beam. As a result, the length of the beam decreases on the compression side and increases on the tension side. The beam also contains a neutral axis, where the length of the beam is unchanged. There are neither tensile nor compressive stresses acting at the neutral axis. Therefore, beam material is neutral, or unreactive, to the applied load. The beam is under tensile stress on one side of the neutral axis, and compressive stress on the other side. These stresses increase with increasing distance away from the neutral axis, and are highest at the outer surface of the beam. Therefore, beam material further away from the neutral axis deforms more, i.e. changes more in length. The material at the neutral axis is unreactive to bending forces, and in theory can be removed from the beam without affecting its strength.

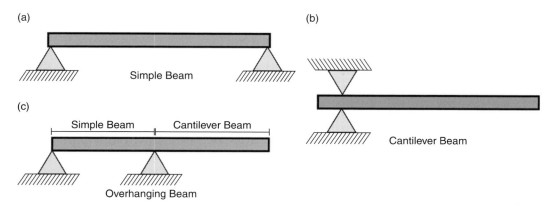

Fig. 3.6 Basic types of beams: (a) simple beam; (b) cantilever beam; (c) overhanging beam.

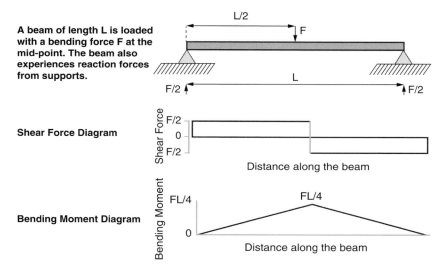

A beam of length L is loaded with a bending force F at the mid-point. The beam also experiences reaction forces from supports.

Shear Force Diagram

Bending Moment Diagram

Fig. 3.7 Mechanics of a beam. Shear force and bending moments' diagrams for a simply supported beam subjected to a single point load acting in the middle. The applied force produces shear forces and bending moments within the beam, which vary along its length. (L = length, F = force).

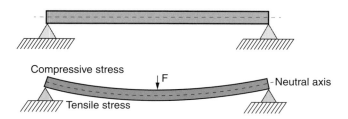

Fig. 3.8 Simple beam theory. A beam tends to change shape when subjected to an applied force. It experiences compressive stress on the side of the applied force and tensile stress on the opposite side. The neutral axis within the beam experiences neither compressive nor tensile stresses. The stresses in the beam increase with increasing distance away from the neutral axis, and are highest at the outer surface of the beam.

Bending II

The effect of cross-sectional geometry on the properties of a beam

Simple beam theory shows that, in bending, stresses are unevenly distributed within a structure; stresses are higher at the outer surface than at the centre of a structure. Therefore, although a structure's strength in axial compression and tension is determined by its cross-sectional area, i.e. mass, a structure's strength in bending is related to its cross-sectional area *and* how the material is distributed about the neutral axis.

The cross-sectional distribution of material in a beam is described mathematically as 'area moment of inertia'. The area moment of inertia quantifies the bending resistance (stiffness) of a given cross-section: the larger the area moment of inertia, the greater the bending resistance and so, the less the stress produced within a structure under a given bending force. Different cross-sectional shapes provide different resistances to bending. Therefore, two beams made of the same material with equal cross-sectional areas, but different cross-sectional shapes would be equally strong in compression and tension, but have different strengths in bending.

Simple beam theory and the principle of area moment of inertia show that structures are more resistant to bending when the cross-sectional material is distributed further away from the neutral axis. Therefore, it is possible that, with careful planning, material in the centre of a beam may be removed without significantly affecting its ability to withstand bending forces. The bending stiffness of a hollow beam is related to the thickness of its walls and the outer diameter; the outer diameter usually has a much greater effect than the thickness of the walls. The main drawback of a hollow beam is that, if it is loaded beyond its strength, it fails more suddenly than a solid beam, as there is less material for a fracture to propagate across.

The cross-sectional geometry of orthopaedic implants determines their bending stiffness. For example, an intramedullary nail has a cylindrical cross-section, therefore its bending resistance is proportional to its radius to the fourth power, whereas a plate has a rectangular cross-section and so its bending resistance is proportional to its thickness to the third power. Also, based on inherent moment of inertia, a hollow nail must be wider than a solid nail for an equal bending resistance. The material properties of implants also affect their bending stiffness, e.g. the stiffness of titanium alloy is about half that of stainless steel, and therefore a titanium plate would have half the stiffness of an identical plate made of stainless steel. However, in general situations, the cross-sectional geometry dominates the material properties in determining bending stiffness, and therefore a titanium plate could be made to be as stiff as stainless steel plate by slightly increasing its thickness (although this is normally not required).

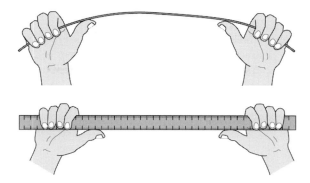

Fig. 3.9 A beam's stiffness depends on the distribution of the cross-sectional material relative to the applied load. A plastic ruler can be bent more easily in one direction than in the other. Although the cross-sectional area of the ruler is constant, its stiffness increases when more material is aligned in the direction of applied force. I-beams in the construction industry take advantage of this concept.

Basic equation for calculating

Cross-section shape	Moment of inertia of area I	Notes
Rectangle 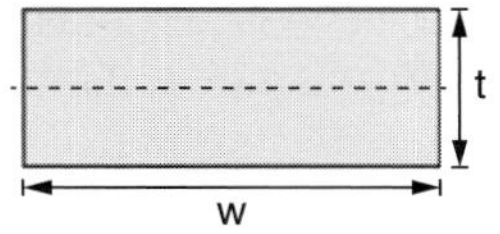	$I = \dfrac{wt^3}{12}$	I is directly proportional to width, w, and thickness, t, to the third power. Doubling t increases I eight fold.
Square 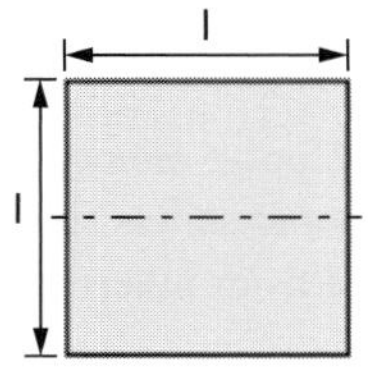	$I = \dfrac{l^4}{12}$	I is directly proportional to length, l, to the forth power. Doubling l increases I sixteen fold.
Circle 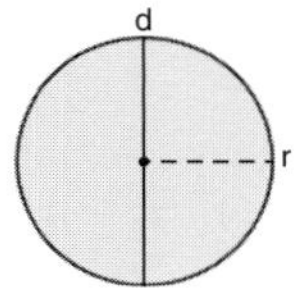	$I = \dfrac{\pi d^4}{64}$, or $I = \dfrac{\pi r^4}{4}$	I is directly proportion to radius, r, to the forth power. Doubling r increases I sixteen fold.
Hollow circle 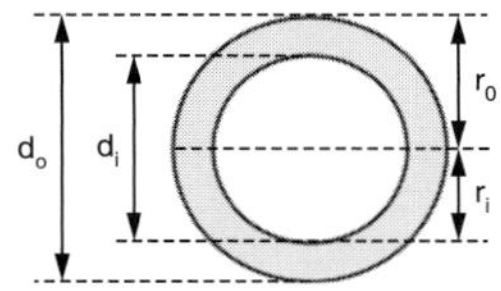	$I = \dfrac{\pi(d_0^4 - di^4)}{64}$ or $I = \dfrac{\pi(r_0^4 - r_1^4)}{4}$	I is directly proportional to $(r_0^4 - r_1^4)$. Doubling r_0^0 and r_1 (i.e keeping thickness constent) increases I sixteen fold.

Fig. 3.10 This table summarises the relationship between common cross-sectional shapes and area moment of inertia (bending stiffness). The neutral axis for all these regular shapes is located at the geometric centre. Structures become more resistant to bending when the cross-sectional material is distributed further away from the neutral axis.

Torsion

A shaft is a solid structure that carries torsional forces. A torsional force is produced when equal and opposite torques are applied to the ends of a structure, causing it to twist along its axis and undergo angular deformation. A torsional force produces complex effects on the shaft. The basic principles of torsional loading are illustrated by a cylindrical shaft. It is assumed that a cylindrical shaft does not experience 'warping' effect when subjected to a torsional force, i.e. its circular cross-section remains circular (whereas the shape of square/rectangular cross-section would change as the shaft is twisted).

Stresses produced in torsion

The stresses produced by torsional forces are shown by drawing squares and diamonds on the surface of the cylinder. A square becomes a parallelogram; this is shear-type deformation (see pages 52–53) and shows that shear stresses are produced in the planes parallel and perpendicular to the axis of the loading. A diamond becomes a rectangle; this is compression- and tension-type deformation and shows that compressive and tensile stresses are acting at 45° to the axis of loading. In fact, torsion produces pure shear in the planes parallel and perpendicular to the longitudinal axis, and tension and compression in planes at other angles. Tensile and compressive stresses are highest at 45° to the longitudinal axis. Tensile and compressive stresses are driven by, and add up to, shear stresses produced by the torsional force.

In the same way as in a simple beam, magnitude of stresses in a shaft also varies along its thickness. A shaft has a neural axis at the centre of its cross-section where no stresses act on the material. Stresses then increase with increasing distance away from the neutral axis, and are highest on the outer surface of the shaft.

Effect of cross-sectional geometry on properties of a shaft

Just as in a simple beam, stresses are non-uniformly distributed within a shaft; stresses are higher at the outer surface than at the centre. Therefore, a structure's torsional strength is also determined by the cross-sectional area *and* how the material is distributed about the neutral axis. A structure develops a higher resistance to torsion as the material is distributed further away from the neutral axis.

The cross-sectional resistance to angular deformation is measured mathematically in terms of 'polar moment of inertia': the larger the polar moment of inertia, the greater the resistance to angular deformation and so less stress is produced within a structure under a given torsional force. Polar moment of inertia (J) is derived from inherent moment of inertia (I) with the following equation:

$$J \, [\mathrm{m^4}] = 2 \times I \, [\mathrm{m^4}]$$

Therefore, polar and inherent moments of inertia essentially represent the same basic measurement: the distribution of material about its neutral axis.

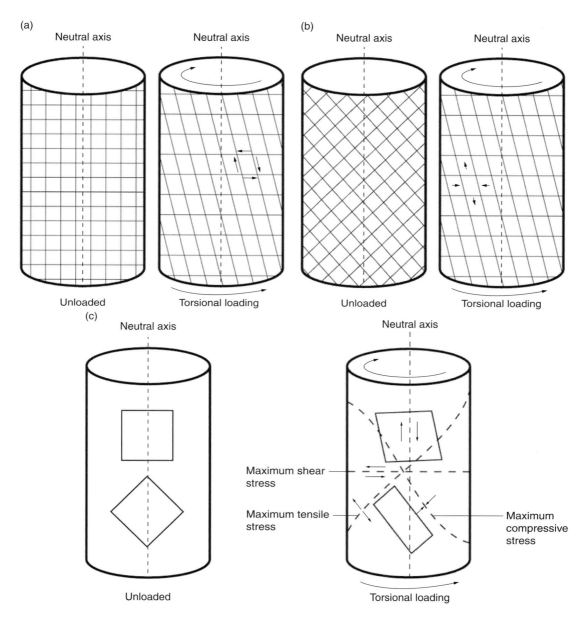

Fig. 3.11a-c Basic principles of torsional loading are illustrated by a cylindrical shaft. A cylindrical shaft maintains a circular cross-section when subjected to a torsional force. (a) The squares drawn on the surface of the cylinder show shear-type deformation. This indicates that torsion generates shear forces and stresses in planes parallel and perpendicular to the axis of loading. If the cylinder is prismatic, i.e. it has a uniform cross-section throughout its length, then all squares along the length of the cylinder become identical parallelograms, indicating that shear stress remains constant along the length of a prismatic shaft. (b) The diamonds drawn on the surface of the shaft show compression- and tension-types of deformation. (c) Torsion therefore produces a complex series of interrelated stresses.

Material and geometric properties of long bones

The musculoskeletal system is subjected to widely variable loads. Bones have evolved into perfect scaffolds for withstanding all four modes of loading. As dynamic structures, bones can change with age and in response to applied loads and have the ability to self-repair. The material and geometric properties of bones are finely adapted to their mechanical functions.

Material properties

Bones consist of two distinct sections: cortical bone on the outside and cancellous bone on the inside. Cortical bone is dense and stiff, and almost wholly supports all the forces. Cancellous bone is much less dense and much more ductile. It is excellent in resisting compressive and shear forces. Overall, bone is a brittle material and is therefore much stronger in compression than in tension.

Geometric properties

Some of the highest stresses in the bones are generated by bending and torsion. The long bones have cross-sectional geometry of a hollow cylinder. This optimises their resistance against bending and torsion, without compromising their strength in compression and tension.

Bones of children and adults can be considered to be made of different materials: the immature bone is much less mineralised and therefore ductile and weak, whereas mature bone is much more mineralised and therefore stiffer and stronger but brittle. Therefore, a change in bone material makes bones stiffer and stronger with age. However, the difference in stiffness and strength of immature bone and mature bone cannot be fully explained by a change in bone composition only. The growing bones also develop more resistant cross-sectional geometry: the expanding diameter of growing bones considerably increases their resistance to bending and torsion. In fact, the relationship of the bone's cross-sectional diameter to length is critical in children. The long bones form lever arms for muscle function, and in children, as the long bones increase in length, there is a compensatory increase in the cross-sectional diameter to maintain strength.

In general, the size of bones in adults seems to be predetermined by genetics and nutrition. However, the thickness of cortical walls is greatly affected by applied loads. Exercise, especially weight training, can significantly increase the cross-sectional area of bones. Muscle contractions generate some of the highest stresses on the bones. Therefore, as resistance exercises increase the size of muscles over time, the underlying bones remodel to develop thicker cortices. Thicker cortices lead to a larger cross-sectional area and area/polar moments of inertia, which strengthen bones for the increased demands. The relationship between muscle function and bone mass is so critical that, throughout the animal kingdom, an individual's total bone mass is a function of its total muscle mass, i.e. lean (and not total) body mass (Table 3.1).

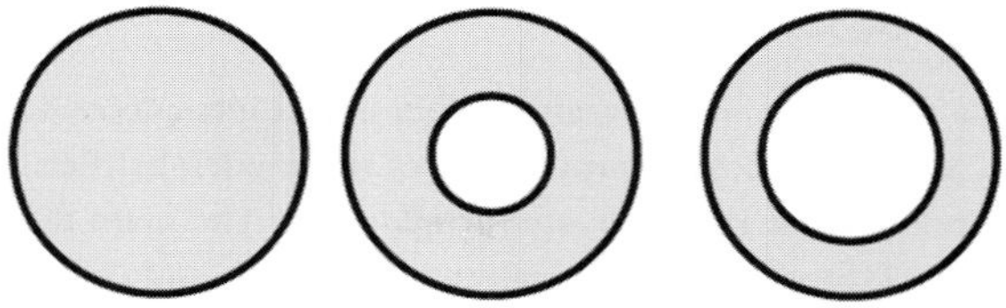

Relative cross-section area	100%	100%	87%
Relative resistance to tensile and compressive loads	100%	100%	87%
Relative resistance to bending and torsional loads	100%	164%	208%

Fig. 3.12 An illustration of the influence of cross-sectional geometry of bone on resistance against the four modes of loading. It is assumed that the bones have identical composition and length.

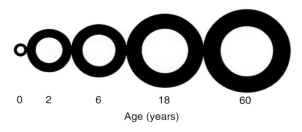

0	2	6	18	60	

Age (years)

Fig. 3.13 This diagram illustrates the change on cortical diameter of the femur with age. In the growing bone, cross-sectional diameter increases with bone length to maintain strength. In the ageing bone, osteoporosis affects the bone material – making it mechanically weaker – but a compensatory increase in bone diameter preserves whole bone strength.

Table 3.1. **Allometry**

Allometry is the study of the relationship between the size of an organism and the size of its body parts. Allometric studies show that, in an animal, the size of bones is proportional to its body mass as follows:

$$\text{Cross-sectional diameter of bone} \propto (\text{body mass})^{0.33}$$
$$\text{Bone length} \propto (\text{body mass})^{0.33}$$

These correlations are confirmed by studies investigating bone dimensions in animals with body mass differing by six orders of magnitude.

Fundamentals of fracture

In mechanics, a fracture is the separation of an object into pieces due to an applied load at a temperature below its melting point. Materials fracture through one of two modes: brittle and ductile. Both modes involve two basic steps of the fracture process: crack initiation and propagation. The main difference between the two modes is in the mechanism of crack progression. All materials are rough and contain defects and cracks at microscopic level. Crack initiation occurs when the applied load leads to sufficient stress in the material to increase the size of a crack. Crack progression in a brittle fracture is associated with little plastic deformation, whereas ductile fracture involves significant plastic deformation. Materials therefore can be labelled as brittle or ductile to describe their performance under load.

Brittle fracture

In brittle fracture, a crack almost always initiates on the surface of the material. It then propagates almost perpendicular to the applied stress, leaving a flat fracture surface. The crack is referred to as 'unstable' as it propagates spontaneously when the stress threshold for crack initiation is reached. There is relatively little energy absorbed in the fracture process. Brittle fracture therefore occurs rapidly with little or no pre-warning. It is usually a catastrophic situation, as there is no opportunity to anticipate an impending fracture or to repair accumulating damage to prevent complete failure.

Cortical bone is a brittle material and sustains brittle fracture. Other brittle materials include ceramics, ice, cast iron and metals at low temperatures. Brittle materials display little plastic deformation before failure and have the tendency to break into many pieces.

Ductile fracture

In ductile fracture, a crack initiates in the substance of the material. The material undergoes extensive plastic deformation at the site of the crack propagation. The crack is referred to as 'stable' as it resists further extension unless increased stress is applied. There is substantial energy absorption in the fracture process. The plastic deformation and incremental fracture progression produce a 'cup and cone' fracture surface.

Most metals are ductile at room temperature. Ductile materials display large deformation before failure and usually break into two main pieces.

Ductile materials are preferred for most engineering applications. Ductile materials are 'tough' as they absorb more energy than brittle materials. They also show warning signs of fracture and therefore present an opportunity to intervene before complete failure. Ductile materials are considered to be forgiving, since their toughness usually allows them to tolerate excessive loads. The properties of ductile materials can also be enhanced through strengthening mechanisms.

Brittle fracture is the commonest mode of fracture of engineering components (even those made from ductile materials). This is because most engineering components undergo fatigue failure, in which the fracture propagates in brittle mode (Table 4.1).

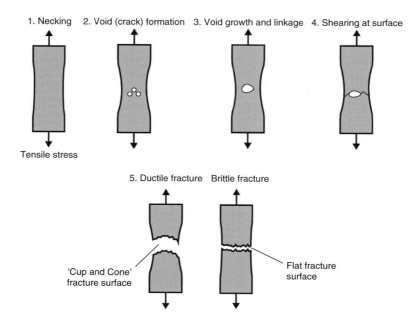

Fig. 4.1 Ductile fracture involves a number of steps. In contrast, brittle fracture occurs rapidly in a single step. Ductile fracture produces a 'cup and cone' fracture surface, whereas brittle fracture creates a flat fracture surface.

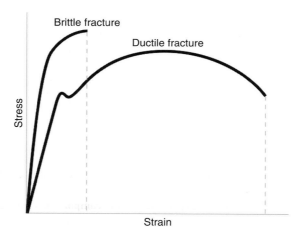

Fig. 4.2 This stress–strain curve shows deformation produced in brittle and ductile fractures. The area under the curves represents energy absorbed by the material until failure. Ductile materials are 'tough' as they absorb more energy than brittle materials.

Table 4.1. **Ductile to brittle transition in metals**

The Titanic was the largest and most advanced ship of its time in 1912. It sank after colliding with an iceberg during its maiden voyage. Steel used to make the Titanic was tested to be adequately tough to withstand all predictable damages. However, steel taken from the wreck of the Titanic showed signs of brittle failure, i.e. a flat fracture surface with very little plastic deformation. The steel was ductile and tough in the tests performed at room temperature, but brittle and weak at sub-zero sea temperatures. Metals show a transition from ductile to brittle failure at low temperatures. Brittle fracture is sudden and catastrophic, and engineering designs now anticipate and prevent brittle failures in all components.

Mechanism of bone fracture

Cortical bone is anisotropic and brittle, although immature cortical bone is more ductile. In common with other brittle materials, cortical bone is strongest in compression, weakest in shear and intermediate in tension. These mechanical properties determine the mechanism and pattern of bone fracture. The forces acting on the bone also determine the pattern and location of fracture in the bone. As bone properties and the forces both determine fracture pattern, the same forces can produce different fracture patterns in mature and immature bones due to their different mechanical properties.

Mechanism of fracture

A bone fracture is a break in the continuity of bone. The bone typically fractures in a brittle mode. There are two phases to the fracture process: initiation and propagation. The fracture usually initiates on the outside surface of the bone, because this is where stresses are usually highest under most loading conditions. The bone surface is not smooth and polished, but is irregular and full of microscopic defects and cracks. There are also localised regions of relative osteopenia in the bone, where normal remodelling process is under way. These factors together form stress concentration points, one of which becomes a fracture initiation site when a crack begins to increase in size. After initiation, the crack grows in size and propagates rapidly until complete failure.

Acute vs fatigue fracture

Acute fracture occurs when the load applied to an object exceeds its ultimate tensile strength. Most bone fractures are acute. A 'pathological' fracture occurs when the strength of bone is reduced (e.g. due to osteoporosis or malignancy) so that it fails below the usual stress threshold.

An object subjected to cyclical or fluctuating loads is susceptible to fatigue or stress fracture. Fatigue fracture results from a load that is below the material's yield or ultimate tensile strength under static load.* The term 'fatigue' describes that fracture that has resulted from a prolonged period of repetitive loading cycles. Although this is an uncommon cause of bone failure, it is the most common cause of failure of engineering structures.

Fatigue failure builds up slowly but occurs suddenly and without warning. The mechanism of fatigue fracture is similar to brittle fracture mode as it occurs rapidly with relatively little plastic deformation, even in normally ductile materials. The fracture similarly propagates perpendicular to the applied tensile load.

The S–N curve
The *S–N* curve represents the material's performance under cyclical loads. It plots stress amplitude (*S*) against the number of cycles to failure (*N*). Materials fall into two categories, based on whether or not they have a fatigue limit.
- *Fatigue limit.* If stress amplitude is reduced below a particular threshold, fatigue failure will not occur for an infinite number of cycles.
- *No fatigue limit.* Fatigue failure will eventually occur irrespective of stress amplitude level (Table 4.2).

---

* The other mechanical process that can cause a material to fail below its yield strength is creep – see pages 22–23.

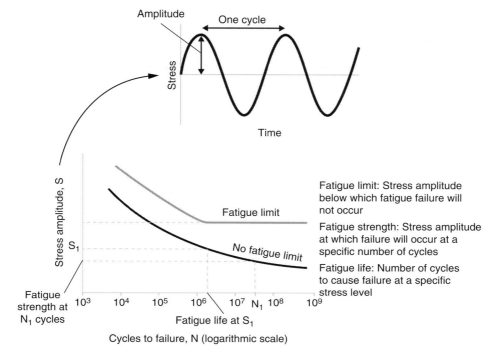

Fig. 4.3 The *S–N* curve represents materials' fatigue properties. It shows that the number of cycles a material can withstand without failure depends on stress amplitude. Some materials show a fatigue (or endurance) limit, e.g. iron and titanium alloys, whereas other materials eventually fail no matter how low the stress amplitude. The study of fatigue failure, especially high-cycle fatigue failure, is a relatively new field (since the age of the steam engine), as in the distant past machines did not go fast enough to develop millions of stress cycles. It is of increasing interest in orthopaedics, as the patients receiving permanent implants are increasingly younger and more active, so fatigue failure is becoming more important.

Table 4.2. **Fatigue properties of bone**

Bone has interesting fatigue properties. *In-vitro* experiments show that bone does not have a fatigue limit and is susceptible to fatigue failure at even small stress amplitudes, given an adequate numbers of cycles. *In-vivo* bone, however, has the capacity to repair, and any fatigue-related micro-damage stimulates bone remodelling. Fatigue failure of bone only occurs when the rate of micro-damage exceeds the rate of remodelling. Therefore, fatigue failure of *in-vivo* bone is related to stress amplitude and frequency of loading.

Patterns of bone fractures I

A load applied to bone produces stress in all directions. The fracture occurs along the weakest plane, which is normally the plane of maximum shear or tensile stress.

A tensile load produces transverse fracture that is perpendicular to the plane of loading. This plane experiences the highest tensile stress, and a crack on this plane separates and propagates into a fracture.

A compressive load on the bone produces oblique fracture. The cortical bone is strong in compression, and fracture occurs along the plane of highest shear stress. A compressive force, as a vector quantity, can be resolved into its rectangular components; the component at 45° is the maximum fraction of the applied force (see pages 52–53 for details). This plane in bone is under the highest shear stress and therefore fails, producing a short oblique fracture that is at approximately 45° to the plane of loading.

A bending load (i.e. three-point bending) can result in a simple transverse fracture or a 'butterfly' fragment. The bending load produces tensile stress at one cortex of the bone and compressive stress at the opposite cortex. The bone is weaker in tension than compression; therefore fracture initiates at the cortex under tensile stress and propagates across to produce a transverse fracture. At the same time, the opposite cortex under compressive stress can also fail independently, initiating an oblique fracture line that joins the transverse fracture line. This leads to fracture comminution and a 'butterfly' fragment, which increases in size with the amount of axial loading (i.e. compression). Four-point bending produces a segmental fracture of the bone.

A torsional load produces spiral fracture. The torsional load generates a complex series of interconnected stresses in different planes: shear stress is maximum at planes parallel and perpendicular to the longitudinal axis to the bone, and tensile and compressive stresses are maximum at 45° (see pages 58–59 for details). Tensile and compressive stresses are driven by shear stresses produced by the torsional load. A small surface crack on the plane of maximum tensile stress begins to increase in size and propagates through to the core and the circumference of the bone, in a spiral pattern following the 45° planes of maximum tensile stress. Shear stress is ultimately responsible for fracture initiation, since maximum tensile stress is driven by shear stress.

The average angle of spiral fracture to the longitudinal axis of bone in experimental studies is between 30° and 40°. In clinical experience, the spiral fracture angle varies widely between 20° to 90°. The difference between experimental and clinical observations is because in reality fracture progression is distorted by bone anisotropy, moments caused by contraction of muscles attached along the length of bone and bony appendages. In addition, an actual torsional injury is usually associated with a bending moment, which limits the progression of the fracture along the length of the bone.

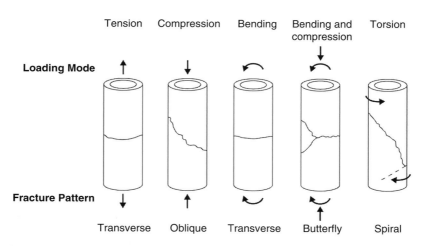

Fig. 4.4 Basic patterns of bone fracture according to loading mode.

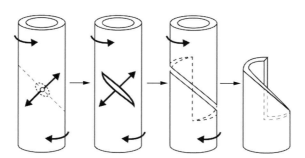

Fig. 4.5 A butterfly fragment fracture pattern is produce by a combination of bending and compressive loads. The bending load initiates a transverse fracture at the cortex under tensile stress, and the compressive load initiates an oblique fracture at the opposite cortex. The two fracture lines meet and a further oblique fracture line breaks off the butterfly fragment.

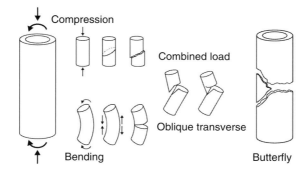

Fig. 4.6 A spiral fracture pattern is produced by a torsional load. The fracture initiates on the plane of maximum tensile stress, and propagates along the planes of maximum tensile stress. A bending moment finally divides the bone.

Patterns of bone fractures II

Immature bones in children have mechanical properties different from those of mature bones in adults. Therefore, there are variations in fracture patterns in children. Immature bones are weaker, but more ductile than mature bones. They have a thicker and firmer periosteum, which acts as a shield around the bone. The bone-periosteum unit has considerably more strength than the immature bone singly, and the periosteum also limits fracture displacement. The periosteum supplies nutrients to the bone and is more metabolically active in children; therefore paediatric fractures unite more rapidly. Immature bones contain physes (growth plates) that determine bone growth and rate of fracture remodelling. The physes can be involved in fractures, which can potentially lead to long-term bone growth disturbances.

A compressive load can produce a torus or 'buckle' fracture in children. This type of fracture typically occurs in the metaphyseal region of long bones. Immature cortical bone is more porous and less dense than mature bone, and so is weak under compressive stress. Therefore, bone cortex under compressive load sustains a local fracture, which does not propagate to the opposite cortex due to the ductile nature of the bone.

A bending load can lead to a greenstick fracture in children. A greenstick fracture is where one bone cortex is broken and the fracture propagates to the opposite cortex, but does not completely disrupt it. This fracture pattern reflects the ductile nature of paediatric bone. The fracture initiates at the cortex under tensile stress, but the opposite cortex under compressive stress undergoes plastic deformation. After initiation, the fracture propagates *longitudinally* along the bone until all the imposed energy is absorbed. The resulting fracture pattern is similar to how an actual greenstick breaks.

A paediatric bone can be so ductile that it can undergo pure plastic deformation, without sustaining a fracture. The adult bone is brittle and does not experience significant plastic deformation; the energy transmitted to the bone dissipates mainly in the form of fracture. However, immature bone is much more pliable and can plastically deform to absorb the applied energy. As plastic deformation absorbs much more energy than brittle failure, bones that have undergone plastic deformation are uncommonly also fractured. Plastic deformation typically occurs under bending load.

Paediatric fractures are managed differently to fractures in adults. The periosteum contributes significantly to fracture stability. Most fractures in children are managed conservatively. Fractures are usually surgically treated only if there is: significantly mal-alignment; significant displacement in a fracture that involves the physis or joint; or if the fracture is unstable. These fractures are stabilised with temporary fixation devices wherever possible (Table 4.3).

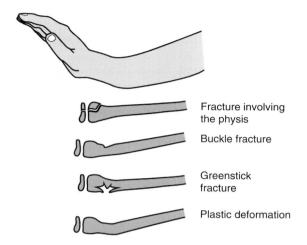

Fracture involving
the physis

Buckle fracture

Greenstick
fracture

Plastic deformation

Fig. 4.7 Variation in fracture patterns in children. Fracture types only seen in children are shown in an illustration of the distal radius.

Table 4.3. **Factors that determine remodelling potential of fractures in children**

Factor	Effect on remodelling of fracture
Skeletal maturity	The younger the child, the greater the remodelling potential of the fracture.
Bone fractured	Different bones have different potential to remodel. Generally, bones in the upper limb have higher remodelling potential than bones in the lower limb. Upper limb fractures around the elbow have a limited remodelling potential. Lower limb fractures around the knee have the greatest remodelling potential.
Site of fracture	Fractures in the metaphyseal region have higher remodelling potential than fractures in the diaphyseal region. This is because the metaphysis undergoes osteogenesis and remodelling as part of normal bone growth.
Plane of deformity	Angulation remodelling potential is inversely related to the distance between the fracture and the nearest joint. Angulation remodelling is highest in the plane of the greatest movement of the joint, e.g. remodelling is highest for volar or dorsal angulation of fractures around the wrist. Remodelling potential for translation and shortening is multifactorial and related to the first three factors. Rotational remodelling potential is very limited.

Patterns of bone fractures III

The previous sections have looked into how bone fracture patterns are determined by the hierarchical structure of the bone, and the applied forces. Here is a summary.

- *Material properties.* Cortical bone is anisotropic and brittle. Therefore, it fractures through brittle mode. The fracture starts on the surface of the bone on a plane of highest shear or tensile stress. It then propagates rapidly, permitting little plastic deformation of bone. Immature cortical bone is more ductile and shows greater plastic deformation and variations in fracture patterns.
- *Structural properties.* Long bones are hollow cylindrical tubes. Bending and torsional loads are mainly concentrated on the peripheral sections. Therefore, fracture starts on the outer surface of the bone. As the bones are hollow, there is less material for the fracture to propagate across.
- *Loading mode.* The type of forces applied determine fracture pattern.

There are two additional physical factors that further influence the pattern of bone fractures.

Arrangement of bones

Bones are just one of the building blocks of the body. Forces are applied to a person rather than to an individual bone. The internal arrangement of bones and other structures also affects the sequence and patterns of fractures of bones. The 'polo mint concept' illustrates the significance of this 'higher-order' arrangement. According to this concept, a ring-like structure, such as a polo mint, usually does not break in only one place but in at least two or more places. Therefore, when bones are arranged into a ring-like structure, e.g. the pelvic ring or the ring formed by the forearm bones in children, it is uncommon for one bone to be fractured in isolation. Therefore, the other bones, joints and soft tissues must be assessed for occult injuries such as fractures, dislocations or ligament sprains. Many fracture classifications are based on the sequence of fractures of bones in close arrangements, e.g. Lauge–Hansen classification of ankle fractures. Therefore, the pattern of bones fracturing is also determined by the relative arrangement of the bones.

Fracture mechanics

The surface of the bone is uneven and contains defects and cracks at microscopic level. When a material is loaded and the stress in the material reaches a specific threshold, one of the defects increases in size and the fracture ensues. It is a fundamental physical occurrence that only *one* of the defects increases in size to produce a complete fracture instead of multiple defects growing into incomplete fractures. This is because bone is brittle and a propagating fracture keeps the stress in the surrounding areas of the material below the threshold for initiating another fracture. Therefore, energy imparted to the bone propagates one failure point to the end before initiating the next failure point. This concept is illustrated in a paper-tearing experiment.

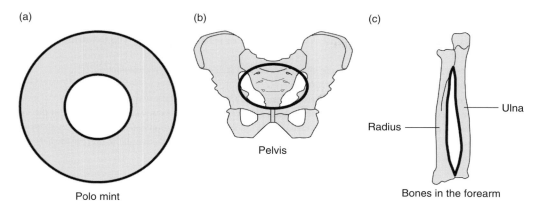

Fig. 4.8 The polo mint concept. (a) A polo mint usually does not break in just one place but instead in two or more places. Similarly, ring-like structures, e.g. the pelvic ring (b) or the ring formed by the forearm bones in children (c), usually do not break in one place only. An obvious injury disturbing the ring should alter to other associated occult injuries, such as fractures of other bones forming the ring or ligament sprains. (In adults, the 'polo mint concept' is less relevant to the injuries of the bones of the forearm.)

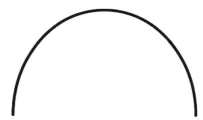

Fig. 4.9 When a strand of dry, uncooked spaghetti is bent, it almost always breaks at two or more places. Uncooked spaghetti is a brittle material, and breaks with flat fracture surfaces. When the spaghetti strand is bent and a weak point breaks, there is a momentary surge in the stress levels along the length of the strand that leads to 'cascade fracturing' at the next weak point, and so on. It may be that a fracture of a bone that is part of a ring also produces excessive stresses at other points in the ring. As the bones forming the ring are relatively fixed in position, increased stresses lead to a cascade injury.

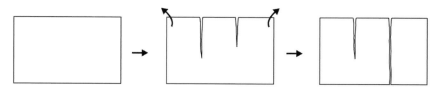

Fig. 4.10 Paper-tearing experiment: Take a plain piece of paper and partially tear it in two places. Then, holding the piece of paper at the edges, try to tear it into three pieces – this would not be possible. The stress produced by the tensile forces propagates one stress raiser to complete failure, instead of simultaneously propagating both stress raisers. This fundamental principle of fracture mechanics also determines patterns of injuries in the musculoskeletal system.

Stress raisers

Stress raisers are geometric flaws normally present on the surface or within a structure. The following are examples of stress raisers:

- *Macroscopic discontinuities*: Voids, notches, threads, sharp corners and sudden changes in cross-section.
- *Microscopic flaws*: Cracks, pores, pits and surface scratches.

When a structure is loaded, these irregularities raise stress in the material in two ways.

- The defects cause a reduction in the area over which the load is distributed, which increases the average stress in the material.
- Stress also concentrates around the tip(s) of defects. The scale of local stress magnification depends on the size, shape and orientation of defects, i.e. different defects have a different stress concentration factor. In general, the sharper the defect, the more severe the stress concentration. Stress raisers often become fracture initiation sites.

Stress raisers therefore significantly reduce the strength of a structure.

Fatigue life

A fatigue fracture always starts at a stress raiser. The number and geometry of stress raisers in a material are critical in determining the load and number of cycles to fatigue failure. Therefore, fatigue life of a structure can be increased by reducing the number and size of stress raisers.

Orthopaedic implants are designed, manufactured and implanted into patients with precautions to minimise stress raisers introduced:

- *Design factors*: Implants are designed to have optimal geometry with the aim to avoid sharp surface discontinuities.
- *Manufacturing aspects*: Materials for implants are carefully selected in terms of their fatigue tolerance and, where possible, further treated to increase their fatigue resistance. Polishing implants at the end of machining operations removes scratches and grooves introduced during the manufacturing process.
- *Surgical technique*: Implants are handled and inserted with techniques that minimise surface scratches.

Orthopaedic procedures can also produce discontinuities in the bone that affect its overall strength. These can be divided into two types:

- *Stress raisers*: A defect, e.g. screw/pin hole, in the bone reduces its strength. There is a direct relationship between the size of the defect and reduction in bone strength. A hole that is one-third of bone diameter reduces bone strength to about 50% of intact bone. The reduction in strength is less if the defect is filled in with another material, e.g. screw or bone graft, than if left unfilled. The stress raiser effect of the defect reduces with time due to bone remodelling. The sharp change in the cross-sectional stiffness at the junction of the end of a prosthesis and bone also creates a stress raiser. A fracture is more likely to initiate in this region if the bone is loaded unexpectedly.
- *Open section defects*: These defects are longer than the bone's diameter, e.g. a bone window for infection or biopsy, and also dramatically reduce bone strength.

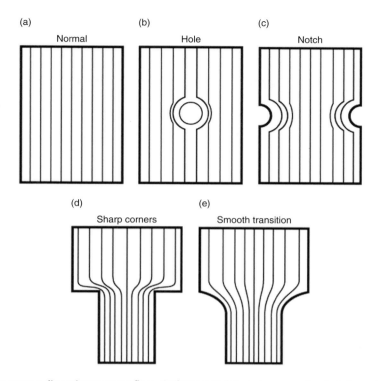

Fig. 4.11 Stress raisers cause a disruption to stress flow, similar to a rock in a stream causing turbulence to water flow. (a) A structure is strongest when stress is uniformly distributed. Stress raisers, such as (b) holes, (c) notches, (d) sharp corners and (e) transition zones, cause local concentration of stress to several times the average stress level in the material.

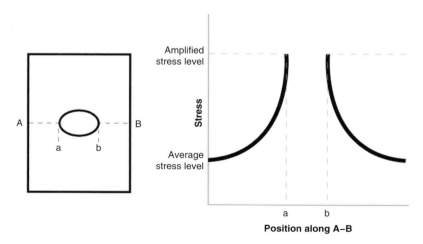

Fig. 4.12 This graph shows that stress is magnified at the tip of a defect and returns to baseline within a distance of three times the diameter of the defect from the tip. Therefore, larger defects affect a wider local area. The impact of a stress raiser on a structure's strength is highlighted when trying to tear open, for example, a bag of peanuts. It is very difficult to split an intact thin sheet of plastic, but a small 'tear here' defect makes the bag much easier to open. The weakening effect of a stress raiser is more significant in a brittle material than a ductile material, and is particularly marked in torsion. (Diagram adapted from Callister, WD (2007). *Material Science and Engineering: An Introduction.* New York: Wiley, with permission from John Wiley & Sons, Inc.)

Corrosion

Corrosion is the deterioration of a structure by chemical reaction with its environment. It is a natural process that occurs because highly reactive materials want to achieve a more stable state as a compound. However, corrosion is a problem, as it removes surface material and creates stress raisers, and therefore reduces the load-carrying capacity of the structure. Corrosion can also induce fatigue failure of a structure under cyclical loading. The biological environment can be very corrosive to foreign material, and corrosion is one of the major processes that lead to implant failure.

As corrosion is a chemical process, it is not described as a mechanical property of a material. Instead, materials are usually described in terms of being immune, resistant or susceptible to corrosion. Metals are particularly susceptible to corrosion. Deterioration of ceramics and polymers is usually analysed as degradation rather than as corrosion.

Types of corrosion

Corrosion is commonly classified according to the appearance of the structure undergoing corrosion or the circumstances in which corrosion occurs. The following are clinically important types:
- Uniform/ general corrosion evenly affects the whole surface area of the structure.
- Localised corrosion is concentrated over a small surface area. This is further divided according to the appearance of the corroding area.
  - Pitting corrosion produces cavities (pits and cracks) on the surface.
  - Crevice corrosion occurs in isolated areas (crevices) that are usually shielded from the environment, e.g. under screw heads if screws are not fully tightened into a plate.
  - Filiform corrosion affects in a random thread-like pattern.
- Galvanic corrosion occurs when two metals with significantly different electrochemical potentials have a physical or electrical contact with a common environment.
- Erosive corrosion occurs where a flowing corrosive fluid damages the structure.
- Fretting corrosion occurs between two surfaces in relative motion. The rate of damage is accelerated because the relative motion between the surfaces removes the corroded layer of material, exposing fresh material for further corrosion (see pages 84–85).

Protection against corrosion

Corrosion prevention is a key consideration when designing engineering components. Materials that have less tendency to corrode are utilised wherever possible. Metals usually form a layer of oxide on the surface, which protects them against corrosion. The protective oxide is ineffective in steel (rust), as it is non-cohesive and peels off, exposing underlying layers to the environment. It is very effective in other metals, such as stainless steel, cobalt–chrome and titanium. Externally used components can be painted or have other surface treatments (e.g. coated with a less reactive material) to prevent water getting to the layer susceptible to corrosion (Table 4.4).

Table 4.4. **Basic chemistry**

Corrosion occurs when the combination of a material (usually a metal) and its environment results in the formation of an electrochemical cell. Corrosion involves an electrochemical reaction that consists of two chemical half-reactions: oxidation and reduction. In the oxidation process, an atom gives up electrons, and in the reduction process, an atom gain electrons. The site in a material where oxidation takes place is referred to as the anode and where reduction occurs is referred to as the cathode. The positive ions at the anode leave the surface for the surrounding environment as corrosion products, e.g. as oxides or hydroxides. The free electrons left behind travel to the site of the cathode through a conductive pathway. At the cathode, the free electrons react with positive ions available in the environment, which restores the electric balance of the circuit. Corrosion therefore is the electrochemical oxidation of a material.

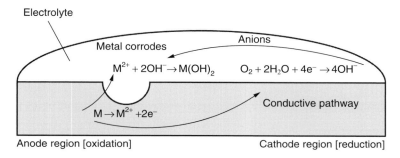

Fig. 4.13 Corrosion reaction requires four essential conditions: an anode, a cathode, a direct electrical connection between the anode and cathode, and an electrolyte (containing dissolved positive ions). In nature, air is the most common electrolyte. In the biological environment, salt solutions (e.g. NaCl) act as the electrolyte medium.

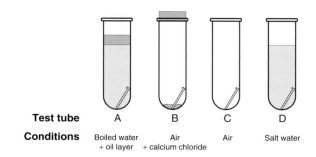

Fig. 4.14 An experiment to show that corrosion requires oxygen and water. Each test tube contains a nail made of iron. Nails in test tubes A and B do not rust. In test tube A, boiled water contains no oxygen, and an oil layer prevents the diffusion of new oxygen. In test tube B, calcium chloride absorbs moisture from the air. The nail in test tube C rusts at a normal rate, due to the presence of air containing oxygen and moisture. The nail in test tube D rusts at an accelerated rate – salt water is an electrolyte (NaCl) solution that conducts ions and therefore speeds up corrosion.

Biological process of bone fracture healing

The aim of the fracture healing process is to reconstruct the broken cortical bone. This healing process begins immediately after a fracture and there are two types: primary (cortical) and secondary (callus) bone healing. Both healing methods involve three basic phases: inflammation, repair and remodelling. Both methods have a common inflammatory phase, but they then diverge in the repair and remodelling phases.

The inflammatory phase begins with the formation of fracture haematoma. This releases inflammatory and repair cells needed to produce new bone. Granulation tissue bridges the fracture site, providing limited mechanical stability.

Primary (cortical) bone healing

The requirements for primary bone healing are that bone fragments are in direct opposition or have only a small gap between them and are rigidly stabilised. This is referred to as 'anatomical reduction and absolute stability'. These conditions are usually achieved by surgical reduction and internal fixation, e.g. with screws and plates, of fracture.

Bone fragments in direct opposition undergo 'contact' healing – this is where osteoclasts from one bone fragment make tunnels, known as cutting cones, across the fracture into the other bone fragment. New blood vessels and osteoblasts arrive in these tunnels and bridge the fracture with new lamellar bone.

Bone fragments with a small gap (≤ 0.5 mm) undergo 'gap healing' – here the gap size is too big for osteoclasts to cross, so osteoblasts work from one end of the fracture and deposit lamellar bone layer by layer until the gap is bridged.

Bone remodelling gradually restores the normal mechanical properties at the fracture over a period of months and years.

Secondary (callus) bone healing

Secondary bone healing occurs where there is a bigger gap between bone fragments and some controlled motion at the fracture site. This is referred to as 'relative stability'. These conditions exist when a fracture is managed conservatively, e.g. in a cast, or internally fixed with implants that provide relative stability, e.g. an intramedullary nail.

There are two stages to the repair process:

- *Soft callus formation.* The granulation tissue is replaced by soft callus consisting of fibroblasts and cartilage, which stabilises the fracture. New bone tissue is laid at the periphery of the fracture site – this is referred to as intramembranous ossification.
- *Hard callus formation.* Intramembranous ossification continues as before. The soft callus within the fracture gap is converted into rigid calcified tissue, i.e. woven bone – this is referred to as enchondral ossification. This process starts at the ends of the fracture and progressively moves towards the centre. Intramembranous ossification bridging the fracture on the outside completes first and enchondral ossification bridging the bone cortices completes afterwards.

Bone remodelling begins after the fracture is fully united with hard callus. It gradually replaces woven bone with lamellar cortical bone over a period of months to years.

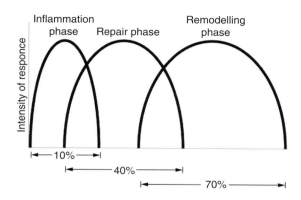

Fig. 4.15 Relative proportion of time involved in the three stages of fracture healing. Fracture healing is a continuous process and there is an overlap between the stages.

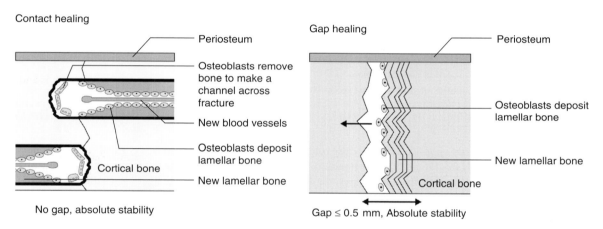

Fig. 4.16 Primary (cortical) bone healing consists of osteoblasts directly depositing lamellar bone. Lamellar bone is the normal bone that consists of parallel layers (lamellae) of collagen fibres.

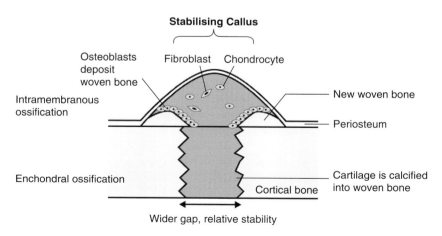

Fig. 4.17 Secondary (callus) bone healing consists of intramembranous and enchondral ossifications. In intramembranous ossification, osteoblasts directly deposit woven bone (without an initial cartilage precursor). In enchondral ossification, osteoblasts form an initial cartilage precursor, which calcifies into woven bone. Long bones normally grow in width by intramembranous ossification, and in length by enchondral ossification. Woven bone consists of randomly organised collagen fibres.

Biomechanical process of bone fracture healing

The biomechanical conditions at the fracture site determine the time involved in fracture healing. The two prerequisites for fracture healing are adequate blood supply and adequate mechanical stability. Primary bone healing can take longer than secondary bone healing if an implant fixed to the bone, in order to rigidly stabilise the fracture, compromises its blood supply. On the other hand, fracture repair through secondary bone healing can also be affected if fracture stability is not optimal.

There is a complex interaction between the mechanical environment and cellular repair processes at the fracture site. The interfragmentary strain theory relates fracture 'strain' to the different types of fracture healing tissues. Strain quantifies a material's deformation in terms of its original length; therefore, interfragmentary strain is described as:

$$\text{Interfragmentary strain } [\%] = \frac{\text{Fracture gap displacement } [mm]}{\text{Initial fracture gap } [mm]} \times 100\%$$

Interfragmentary strain therefore describes the amount of motion at the fracture site. According to the interfragmentary strain theory, different types of fracture healing tissues tolerate different amount of motion at the fracture site. Therefore, interfragmentary strain:

- above 100% would lead to non-union;
- Between 10% and 100% would lead to granulation and fibrous tissue formation;
- Between 2% and 10% would lead to cartilage and enchondral ossification;
- Less than 2% would lead to cortical bone formation.

This explains the biomechanics of primary and secondary bone healing as follows.

Primary (cortical) bone healing

Bone fragments are directly opposed, or are in close contact, so the initial fracture gap is very small. Therefore, bone fragments must be rigidly fixed to prevent any significant motion, which would equate to high strain, since the initial fracture gap is so small. The rigid fixation ensures that interfragmentary strain is less than 2%, leading to primary bone healing.

Secondary (callus) bone healing

A fracture with a wider gap can tolerate more motion at the fracture site and still maintain interfragmentary strain to a reasonable level. Therefore, such fractures only require relative stability.

Fracture stiffness is proportional to the amount of mineralised tissue at the fracture site. The amount of mineralised tissue at the fracture site increases with healing time. When a bone fracture occurs, fracture haematoma provides limited stability to the fracture site. Once the interfragmentary strain is less than 100%, granulation tissue bridges across the fracture gap. This stiffens up the fracture and reduces interfragmentary strain. This, in turn, allows formation of soft callus. The increased cross-sectional diameter from soft callus further increases fracture stiffness and lowers interfragmentary motion. The soft callus is then mineralised into hard callus, and so on. Therefore, a cycle of progressively stiffer tissues forming at the fracture site reduces interfragmentary strain from 100% to less than 2%, and the cortical bone forms.

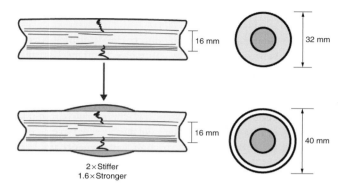

Fig. 4.18 According to the principles of moment of inertia, callus formation at the periosteal surface significantly increases stiffness and strength of the healing bone.

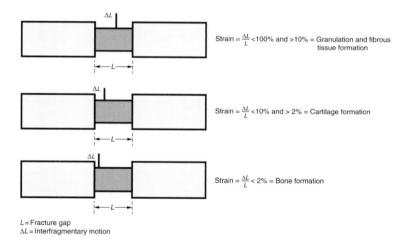

L = Fracture gap
ΔL = Interfragmentary motion

Fig. 4.19 Interfragmentary strain theory. Interfragmentary strain theory states that strain at the fracture site determines the type of fracture healing tissue formed. Primary bone healing takes place when the fracture gap is anatomically reduced and the bone fragments are rigidly stabilised so that interfragmentary strain is less than 2%. Secondary bone healing occurs when the fracture gap is wider and when the bone fragments are relatively stabilised. Secondary bone healing occurs in a cycle of progressively stiffer tissues forming at the fracture site. It requires controlled interfragmentary motion. An unstable fracture (interfragmentary strain >100%) may not heal, despite good callus formation and may develop hypertrophic non-union. A fracture fixed too rigidly or with too wide a fracture gap may not have sufficient interfragmentary strain and may develop delayed union or atrophic non-union.

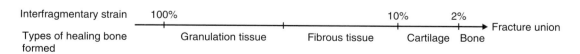

Fig. 4.20 Secondary bone healing

Introduction to biotribology

A force may change the shape and/or state of motion of an object. The deforming effects of force considered so far have been related to the interactions between force and the entire object and mechanisms that result in the failure of the whole structure. This chapter looks into the deforming effects of force on the surface of an object, which in turn are linked with motion parameters of the object. Therefore, in this chapter, deformation and motion of an object are considered together.

Tribology is the study of the interactions between two solid surfaces in relative motion. It deals with friction, wear and lubrication aspects of the interface formed between the solid surfaces. A force acting at the interface produces friction when the surfaces slide over each other. Excessive friction wastes energy and leads to wear of the surfaces. A lubricant acts to reduce friction and wear by creating a slippery film between the surfaces. The thickness of the lubricant film formed between the surfaces determines the effectiveness of the lubrication.

Different interfaces require a different balance of friction, wear and lubrication. High friction is required between foot and ground for walking and in brakes, whereas low friction is desirable between the components of a car engine. Similarly, wear facilitates brushing teeth and is useful when writing with a pencil, but can also be harmful and lead to the breakdown of mechanical components such as gears. The principles of tribology are used to optimise the performance of interacting surfaces in mechanical systems.

Biotribology is the application of tribology to biological surfaces. It is therefore concerned with friction, wear and lubrication aspects of biological systems in sliding contact. Biotribology also includes the study of the interface conditions in prostheses.

Synovial joints are much more complex than general engineering articulations. In addition, biological loading conditions are intense and hugely variable. It is estimated that in a young person, a typical synovial joint undergoes approximately 4700 to 5400 loading cycles everyday and that a typical synovial joint undergoes more than 10^8 loading cycles in an 80-year lifespan. Biotribology provides an insight into the functional conditions of synovial joints, and how they maintain their remarkable performance over prolonged periods of time. This understanding helps to guide the design and development of bearing surfaces of prosthetic joint replacements. This chapter looks into principles of biotribology as applied to synovial joints and prosthetic joints.

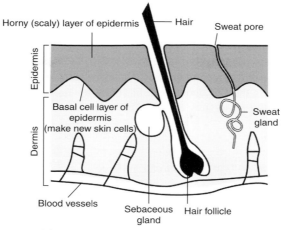

(a) The components and layers of the skin.

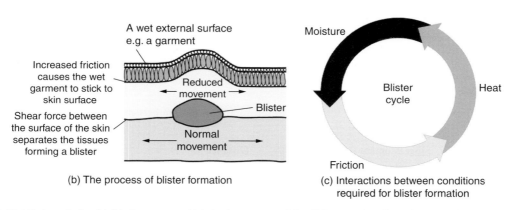

(b) The process of blister formation

(c) Interactions between conditions required for blister formation

Fig. 5.1 Biotribology deals with friction, wear and lubrication aspects of the sliding interface formed between biological surfaces. A key interface in the body is between the skin and the physical world. A sebum (lubricant) film present on the surface reduces friction and wear of the skin. Friction blisters develop when lubrication is not sufficient for the interface conditions. These are almost exclusively confined to humans, and are most common on hands and feet, which are involved in performing repetitive motions. Friction blisters occur when temperature and moisture around the skin are excessively raised (e.g. due to socks on the feet). Higher local temperatures lead to excessive sweat, which is a less effective lubricant than sebum. This leads to higher friction between the skin and the external surface. Higher friction at the interface limits movement at the skin surface, whilst the normal movement between the deeper layers of the skin is preserved. The shear force produced between the layers of the skin creates a void that is filled with fluid to form a blister. The fluid cushions the deeper layers and protects them from trauma. Epidermal blisters typically are filled with serous fluid, whereas dermal blisters are usually blood filled due to the associated injury to blood vessels.

Friction

Friction is a force that resists relative movement between two surfaces in contact. Friction occurs because no surface is absolutely smooth at the microscopic scale, and asperities (microscopic projections) on one surface interact with asperities on the opposite surface to resist motion. Static friction is the force required to initiate motion, and dynamic friction is the force required to maintain motion between contacting surfaces. Friction is always parallel to the contacting surfaces and opposite to the direction of motion. It can produce deformation, wear and heat, which can change the properties of the contacting surfaces, e.g. when polishing a surface.

Friction equation

Friction is directly proportional to the load applied to the surfaces:

$$\text{Friction} \propto \text{Load}$$
$$\therefore \text{Friction [N]} = \mu \times \text{Load [N]}$$
$$\text{and } \mu = \frac{\text{Friction[N]}}{\text{Load[N]}}$$

μ is the 'coefficient of friction' of the interface and is the ratio between friction and load. It have no units. It indicates how much force per unit load is required to initiate sliding motion between two surfaces. The coefficient of friction depends on the roughness of interacting surfaces, and different interfaces have a different coefficient of friction. Friction is directly proportional to the coefficient of friction.

Friction does not depend on the contact area and sliding speed of the two surfaces. Therefore, the contact area between the surfaces can be increased to reduce pressure without increasing the friction.

Frictional torque

Linear motion between surfaces leads to friction; however, rotational motion between surfaces leads to friction and frictional torque:

$$\text{Since Moment [Nm]} = \text{Force [N]} \times \text{Distance [m]}$$
$$\therefore \text{Frictional torque [Nm]} = \text{Friction [N]} \times \text{Distance from centre of rotation [m]}$$

Frictional torque increases with the diameter, i.e. the moment arm, of the rotating object, but friction is unaffected by an increase in the contacting surface area. The wear of surfaces in rotational relative motion is directly related to frictional torque.

Friction and frictional torque equations assume that there is no lubricant present between the contacting surfaces.

Friction in fluids

Friction also resists movement between different layers in a fluid. The resulting internal resistance to flow of fluid is described as viscosity, i.e. the thickness of fluid. Low viscosity fluids are thin, e.g. water, and high viscosity fluids are thick, e.g. honey. Fluid viscosity provides lubrication between surfaces.

Friction and joints

In terms of biotribology, the functional components of a synovial joint are bone, articular cartilage and synovial fluid. Healthy synovial joints experience very low friction because the cartilage-on-cartilage interface has an extremely low coefficient of friction and synovial fluid provides lubrication. Therefore, synovial joints experience minimum wear throughout life.

Friction and wear are significantly higher in the replacement joints, because the coefficient of friction of replacement materials is a magnitude higher than the cartilage-on-cartilage interface (Table 5.1).

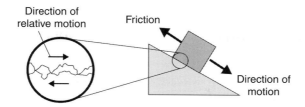

Fig. 5.2 Friction is a force that resists relative movement between two solid surfaces. It only exists when the surfaces are in contact. All surfaces are rough at the molecular scale, so two interacting surfaces are actually in contact at only a very few points, i.e. the 'real' contact area between surfaces is a very small fraction (0.0001%) of the 'apparent' contact area. Therefore, the force applied to the surfaces is acting over a very small area. The high pressures generated deform the contacting points (asperities) and weld them together. Frictional force arises from sliding surfaces breaking and forming bonds between asperities. As the force acting at the interface increases, more opposing asperities make contact, which increases friction.

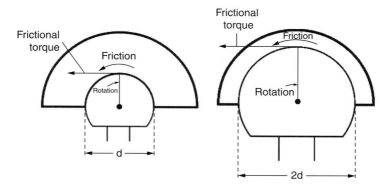

Fig. 5.3 In total hip replacement, for the same bearing combination, a larger diameter femoral head produces a higher frictional torque than a smaller diameter femoral head. Friction between the bearing surfaces is unaffected by the increasing contacting area. Wear of the bearing surfaces is directly related to frictional torque; therefore a larger diameter femoral head produces more wear.

Table 5.1. **Coefficients of friction of different interacting surfaces**

Contacting surfaces	Typical coefficient of friction
Metal on metal (dry)	0.41
Metal on metal (lubricated)	0.06
Teflon on Teflon	0.04
Ice on ice	0.03
Cartilage on cartilage	0.005

Wear

Wear is the progressive removal of material from a contacting surface due to relative motion between two surfaces. It can be measured in terms of depth, i.e. linear wear, or as volume, i.e. volumetric wear, which is more accurate. Wear can also be measured in terms of weight, but volume provides a truer picture when contacting surfaces are made of materials of different densities. Wear is usually detrimental, as it leads to increased mechanical loading and also fatigue failure of the bearing surfaces. The rate of wear is strongly influenced by the interface conditions.

Wear equation

Volume of wear is directly proportional to load and sliding distance between two surfaces.

$$\text{Volume of wear} \propto \text{Load} \times \text{sliding distance}$$

$$\therefore \text{Volume of wear } [\text{mm}^3] = K \, [\text{mm}^3/\text{N mm}] \times \text{Load } [\text{N}] \times \text{Sliding distance } [\text{mm}]$$

$$\text{and,} \quad K \, [\text{mm}^3/\text{N mm}] = \frac{\text{Volume of wear } [\text{mm}^3]}{\text{Load } [\text{N}] \times \text{Sliding distance } [\text{mm}]}$$

K is the 'coefficient of wear' and describes the volume of wear per unit load and sliding distance, i.e. 'wearability' of a given combination of materials. Therefore, the volume of wear is also directly proportional to the coefficient of wear of the interacting surfaces.

In addition to the load and motion variables, wear is also related to the properties of the contacting surfaces. Wear increases with surface roughness and decreases with surface hardness. If the two surfaces are of different materials, wear increases with the difference between the hardness of two surfaces, i.e. the softer material wears more. In other words, when the two surfaces have different hardness, wear depends on the hardness of the softer surface. In the wear equation, the coefficient of wear reflects the hardness of the softer material.

Wear and joints

In synovial joints, wear leads to failure of articular cartilage and development of osteoarthritis. The term 'osteoarthritis' is a misnomer, as it implies that the primary process is inflammatory, whereas there is only degenerative wear of the joint.

The following are some examples of methods of reducing articular cartilage wear:

- A reduction in body weight reduces the overall joint load.
- After an intra-articular fracture, restoration of the joint surface to minimise intra-articular step, i.e. reducing surface roughness.
- An osteotomy around the knee shifts the load from one compartment to another and therefore modifies wear rate of the compartments.
- An osteotomy around the hip can:
  - improve joint contact area/congruency
  - improve femoral head cover
  - shift normal articular cartilage to a weight-bearing area
  - reduce excessive joint reaction force.

Joint replacement prostheses are produced with highly polished bearing surfaces. Polishing reduces roughness of the bearing surfaces, which minimises excessive wear and also removes any stress raisers that can potentially initiate a fracture.

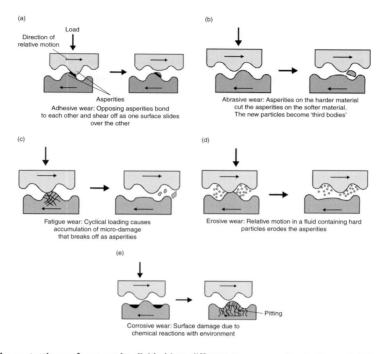

Fig. 5.4a-e **Wear of the contacting surfaces can be divided into different types according to the underlying mechanism producing wear particles**. Mechanical mechanisms include adhesive, abrasive, fatigue and erosive wear. Chemical mechanisms lead to corrosive wear. These mechanisms may occur singly or in combination. (a) *Adhesive wear*: opposing asperities bond to each other and shear off as one surface slides over the other. (b) *Abrasive wear*: asperities on the harder material cut the asperities on the softer material. The new particles become 'third bodies'. (c) *Fatigue wear*: cyclical loading causes accumulation of micro-damage that breaks off as asperities. (d) *Erosive wear*: relative motion in a fluid containing hard particles erodes the asperities. (e) *Corrosive wear*: surface damage due to chemical reactions with environment.

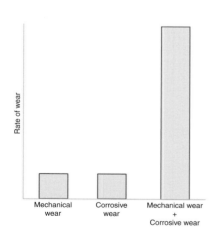

Fig. 5.5 **Wear rate is particularly high when a mechanical type of wear occurs in combination with corrosive wear**. Mechanical wear efficiently removes wear particles produced by corrosive wear, which continually reveals fresh material beneath that in turn corrodes rapidly, and the cycle continues.

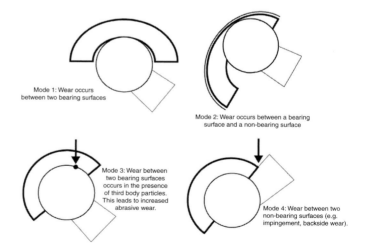

Fig. 5.6 **According to McKellop's classification, wear of artificial joints is divided into four modes**. These four modes of wear are illustrated in bearing surfaces of total hip replacement. Mode 1 represents normally functioning implants, whereas modes 2–4 represent malfunctioning implants. Modes 2–4 can occur singly or in combination, causing massive wear and rapid implant failure.

Lubrication I

A lubricant is a material introduced between two solid surfaces in relative motion in order to reduce friction. Movement between the layers of lubricant and/or a surface and lubricant produces less friction, and therefore surface wear, than movement between the two surfaces alone. The most important property of a lubricant is viscosity. Different interacting surfaces require lubricants with different viscosity. A lubricant may sometimes increase wear, e.g. if it changes mode of wear of the surfaces or traps abrasive particles.

Modes of lubrication

When a lubricant is present between two surfaces, three types of lubrication are possible, depending on the thickness of the fluid film formed during relative motion between the surfaces.

- *Boundary lubrication.* The fluid film between the interacting surfaces is about the same thickness as their surface roughness, so the asperities on the opposing surfaces are in contact. The load on the interface is carried by surface asperities rather than by the lubricant. The interface has a high coefficient of friction, so there is high friction and wear between the surfaces; these can be reduced if a lubricant can adhere to the asperities instead of simply pooling between the asperities.
- *Mixed lubrication.* The fluid film between the two surfaces is slightly thicker than their surface roughness, but there is some contact between the longer asperities on the opposing surfaces. Therefore, the two surfaces are partly in contact and partly separated by the fluid film. The load is shared by the asperities and the fluid film. In comparison with boundary lubrication, this interface has a lower coefficient of friction, so there is lower friction and wear between the surfaces.
- *Fluid film lubrication.* The fluid film completely separates the interacting surfaces. Fluid film lubrication is further divided into two main subtypes.
  - *Elastohydrodynamic lubrication.* The relative motion between the two surfaces maintains a thin layer of fluid film between them. The surfaces, however, are still close enough to cause elastic deformation of the asperities.
  - *Hydrodynamic lubrication.* The relative motion between surfaces maintains a sufficiently thick layer of fluid between them to allow one surface to float above the other. The load is fully supported by the fluid film.

  Motion between the surfaces is essential for achieving and maintaining fluid film lubrication. A change in motion parameters affects the type of fluid film lubrication achieved, if at all. As an example, a machine can have moving parts that experience fluid film lubrication at full function, but not at start-up or shut-down.

The motion conditions between the two solid surfaces determine the type of lubrication regime achieved. The three modes of lubrication can be achieved by a number of different mechanisms, e.g. fluid film lubrication in the synovial joints.

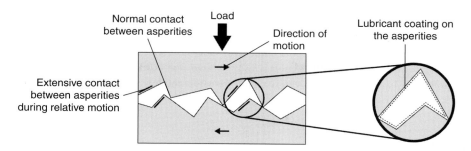

Fig. 5.7 Boundary lubrication. Thickness of fluid film is not sufficient to separate the contacting surfaces. Relative motion between the surfaces results in extensive contact between asperities. However, friction and wear are reduced because the lubricant coats the asperities and the interaction between the chemical compounds in the lubricant on asperities produces less resistance than interaction between 'dry' asperities.

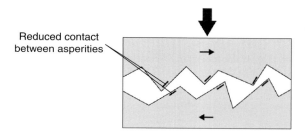

Fig. 5.8 Mixed lubrication. Fluid film between the surfaces is slightly thicker than surface roughness; however, relative motion between the surfaces still results in some contact between longer asperities on opposing surfaces.

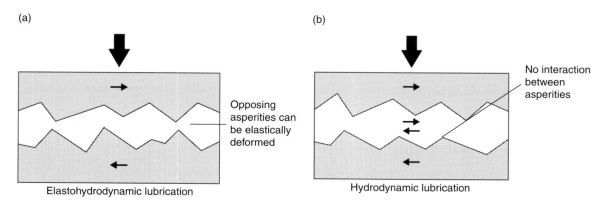

Fig. 5.9 Fluid film lubrication. A continuous layer of fluid film completely separates the interacting surfaces. Fluid film lubrication is divided into two types. (a) Elastohydrodynamic lubrication produces a thin layer of fluid film that separates surface asperities. However, opposing surface asperities can still be elastically deformed; (b) Hydrodynamic lubrication achieves a sufficiently thick layer of fluid film to prevent any type of interaction between opposing asperities. The layers of the fluid film immediately adjacent to each surface travel at the same speed and direction of each surface. The change in direction of relative motion occurs between the layers of fluid, so the surface wear is negligible. Hydrodynamic lubrication occurs when there is sufficient pressure within the lubricant to produce a non-compressible fluid film that is three times thicker than the surface roughness.

Lubrication II

Boundary lubrication is generally the least effective as there is still a significant solid-on-solid contact, and friction and wear at the interface are high; fluid film lubrication is the more desirable as the solid surfaces are fully separated, and friction and wear at the interface are negligible. However, fluid film lubrication is very complex to attain, and interface conditions have to be optimum to achieve this low friction and low wear state of relative motion between surfaces.

The Stribeck curve

The mode of lubrication achieved is determined by three variables:
- viscosity of the lubricant
- speed of relative movement between surfaces
- load acting at the interface.

The Stribeck curve shows the relationship of coefficient of friction to these variables. It shows that boundary lubrication and high coefficient of friction exist when the lubricant is too thin and/or when relative motion between surfaces is too slow for the load acting at the interface. As the lubricant viscosity and/or speed of motion increases or the load decreases, the surfaces begin to move apart, and mixed and fluid film modes of lubrication progressively take effect.

The Stribeck curve also shows that, if the lubricant viscosity remains constant, then the speed of motion must increase with the load to achieve fluid film lubrication.

The Stribeck curve further shows that the coefficient of friction can increase again within fluid film lubrication. This is because drag occurs within the lubricant when the speed of motion between the two surfaces is high.

Synovial fluid as a lubricant

Synovial fluid provides nourishment to the articular cartilage, removes waste products and provides joint lubrication.

Composition. Synovial fluid is produced by the synovial membrane of the joint, and is an ultrafiltrate of blood plasma. It mainly consists of water, hyaluronic acid and proteins, such as albumin.

Lubricant properties. Synovial fluid is a 'shear-thinning' type of fluid – this means that it has a higher viscosity, i.e. is thicker, when still and has lower viscosity, i.e. becomes runnier, when stirred. The Stribeck curve shows that, as the lubricant's viscosity increases, it is able to support more load.

The viscosity of synovial fluid is also proportional to hyaluronic acid concentration, which is essential for its lubrication function. In addition to its lubricant role in the 'dissolved' state, hyaluronic acid also forms complexes with glycoproteins on the surface of the articular cartilage, thereby providing a lubricant coating to the interacting surfaces.

Articular cartilage as a bearing material

Hyaline cartilage lines the bones in a synovial joint. It is a highly organised tissue that consists of cells and extracellular matrix. It forms a low-friction, low-wear bearing material that is viscoelastic, flexible and durable. The different components of articular cartilage help to absorb and distribute the compressive forces experienced by the synovial joint (Table 5.2).

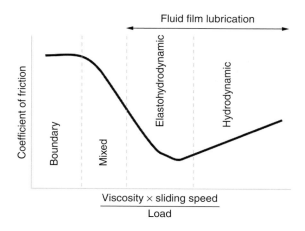

Fig. 5.10 The Stribeck curve. The Stribeck curve shows how the operating conditions at an interface determine the type of lubrication and therefore the coefficient of friction and wear properties of the interface. In boundary lubrication, the coefficient of friction is mainly determined by the properties of interacting surfaces; as in a normal situation of two solid surfaces in direct contact, the coefficient of friction is independent of sliding speed and directly proportional to load. In mixed and fluid film lubrication, the coefficient of friction varies with sliding speed. Just as there is a 'friction equation' and a 'wear equation', the Stribeck curve can be considered to show the 'lubrication equation'.

Table 5.2. **Characteristics of normal synovial fluid in an adult knee joint**

Volume	<3.5 ml
Clarity	Clear
Colour	Colourless/Straw colour
White cell count	<2000/mm^3
Polymorphs	<25%
Gram stain	Negative

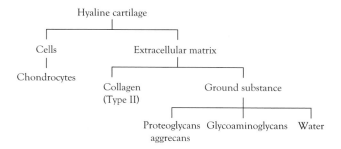

Fig. 5.11 The composition of articular cartilage. Chondrocytes secrete the extracellular matrix components. The relative proportion of different components varies with depth from the articular surface. The thickness of articular cartilage is highly variable; however, its basic composition remains quite constant.

Lubrication of synovial joints

From a biotribology point of view, normal synovial joints have the following functional conditions:

- Articular cartilage forms the two bearing surfaces in relative motion.
- Synovial fluid acts as the lubricant and is present only in small quantities.
- Synovial joints experience large and variable joint reaction forces.
- Synovial joints intermittently are mobile with variable speed of motion.

These are tough operating conditions for lubrication, and are generally opposite to the requirements for fluid film lubrication. However, the articular cartilage and synovial fluid function together to provide a very low coefficient of friction at the interface.

A synovial fluid film exists between the two articular cartilage surfaces at practically all times. The intermittent and relatively low speed of motion of the joints mean that fluid film lubrication cannot always be produced by motion dynamics alone, i.e. the standard mechanisms for elastohydrodynamic and hydrodynamic lubrication. The articular cartilage has the capacity to exude and absorb synovial fluid, much as a sponge can hold and release water. The cartilage-on-cartilage interface therefore has additional mechanisms for achieving fluid film lubrication under different conditions:

- *Weeping lubrication*. If a synovial joint is simply loaded with little or no relative motion between the articular surfaces, the fluid is squeezed out of the cartilage into the joint cavity, thereby maintaining a fluid film between the surfaces. There is a natural limit to this process when a balance between hydrostatic and osmotic pressures is achieved between the two compartments. The fluid returns into the cartilage as the load is eased off.
- *Squeeze film lubrication*: An applied load can also squeeze synovial fluid out from between the two cartilage surfaces. The generated fluid pressure keeps the two surfaces apart. This is considered to be the main lubrication mechanism in shock absorption during high impact situations, e.g. landing on ground after a fall from height.
- *Boosted lubrication*: After prolonged loading, the cartilage absorbs synovial fluid. Cartilage pores are too small for hyaluronic acid. Therefore, the synovial fluid remaining in the joint is more concentrated and has a higher viscosity and load-bearing capacity.
- *Other mechanisms*: Further theories are emerging to explain the maintenance of fluid film lubrication in the synovial joint.

Mixed and boundary lubrication regimes take effect progressively under severe and/or prolonged loading conditions, i.e. when synovial fluid film decreases. The wear of cartilage then depends on its surface properties. The cartilage surface is covered in glycoproteins, which are large molecules and equivalent to surface asperities. The interaction between the glycoproteins on the opposing cartilage surfaces produces a very low coefficient of friction because these are coated with hyaluronic acid or synovial fluid. In addition, cartilage is viscoelastic and can undergo significant deformation before permanent wear.

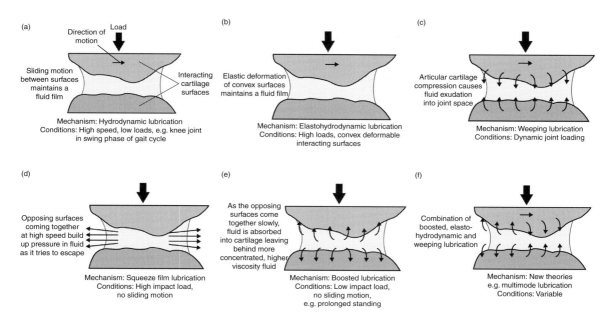

Fig. 5.12 Mechanisms of fluid film lubrication in synovial joints. Different modes of lubrication act at different stages of joint motion. (a) Hydrodynamic lubrication; (b) Elastohydrodynamic lubrication; (c) Weeping lubrication; (d) Squeeze film lubrication; (e) Boosted lubrication; (f) Other mechanisms.

Lubrication of prosthetic joints

The prosthetic joints face the same biotribological challenges as their respective synovial joints, but without the ultra-efficient, variable-mode articular cartilage–synovial fluid lubrication system. The prosthetic bearings do not have a built-in lubricant and only have the articular fluid available for this. The design of bearing surfaces is constrained by functional requirements, such as anatomical, stability and range of motion considerations. Furthermore, the wear particles from prosthetic bearings can interpose between the surfaces and increase wear. Therefore, it is very difficult and complex to achieve satisfactory lubrication between prosthetic bearings, and wear remains a major limitation in their performance.

Wear of total hip and knee replacement prostheses is a particularly significant issue, as these are the two most common joint replacements. Fluid film lubrication is the ultimate in minimising wear between bearing surfaces. In total hip replacement, the ball and socket configuration and motion parameters of bearing surfaces create the possibility of attaining fluid film lubrication. However, a number of other factors also determine if fluid film lubrication is actually achieved.

- *Material of the bearing surfaces.* Polyethylene has a very coarse surface, which does not support fluid film lubrication. In metal on polyethylene combination, wear of polyethylene acetabular cup is managed by using a smaller diameter femoral head that produces a lower frictional torque, e.g. Charnley's 'low frictional total hip arthroplasty' with a 22.5 mm diameter metal head on polyethylene cup, and/or using highly cross-linked polyethylene that has a higher wear resistance. Metals and ceramics have much lower surface roughness; therefore metal on metal and ceramic on ceramic bearing combinations support fluid film lubrication.
- *Diameter of the femoral head.* The likelihood of achieving fluid film lubrication increases as the femoral head diameter increases. Therefore, larger diameter metal on metal and ceramic on ceramic bearing combinations have the highest possibility of achieving fluid film lubrication. The smaller diameter articulations are more likely to experience mixed lubrication.
- *Radial clearance between femoral head and acetabular cup.* The polar bearing articulation allows fluid movement between the bearing surfaces and therefore is the most receptive of fluid film lubrication. However, if the radial clearance is too high, the contact area of bearing surfaces becomes too small, which leads to high wear rates. The congruent bearing articulation has more restricted flow of fluid and equatorial bearing articulation 'locks out' fluid. Therefore, these effects impede support for fluid film lubrication.

The design features and interface conditions of total knee replacement components rule out any significant lubrication between the bearing surfaces. The main biotribological issue in total knee replacement is the wear of the polyethylene tibial insert. This is managed by using components of appropriate design (see pages 120–124) and avoiding using a too thin (<8 mm) tibial insert. In addition, a tibial insert made of highly cross-linked polyethylene has a higher wear resistance than one made of plain polyethylene (Table 5.3).

Table 5.3. **Wear rate of total hip replacement bearing surfaces**

Bearing combination	Typical wear rate per million cycles (mm³)*
Metal on polyethylene	55
Metal on metal	0.6
Ceramic on ceramic	0.16

* The femoral head diameter and joint load are similar in these bearing combinations.

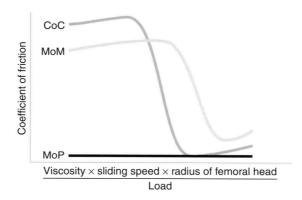

Fig. 5.13 The Stribeck curves for different bearing combinations in total hip replacement. The *x*-axis contains an additional element of the interface: the radius of the femoral head.* The curves show that metal on polyethylene (MoP) bearing combination does not support fluid film lubrication. Metal on metal (MoM) and ceramic on ceramic (CoC) bearing combinations experience a significant reduction in the coefficient of friction as the radius of the femoral head increases. These therefore support fluid film lubrication when femoral head size increases. Metal on polyethylene is a 'hard on soft' bearing combination that experiences high wear rates despite a very low coefficient of friction. Metal on metal and ceramic on ceramic are 'hard on hard' bearing combinations that experience significantly lower wear rates despite having a much higher coefficient of friction.

*The Stribeck curve in Fig. 5.10 (page 89) is for two surfaces in linear motion. When the two surfaces are in rotational relative motion, the *x*-axis has an additional variable, the radius of the rotating object.

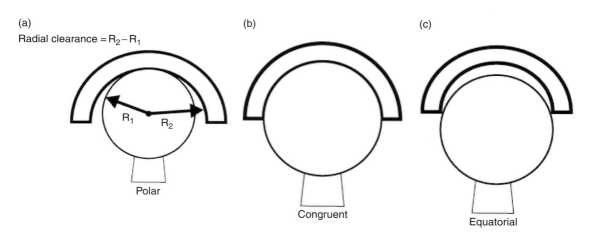

Fig. 5.14 Fluid film lubrication requires radial clearance between the femoral head and acetabular cup. Radial clearance is defined as the difference between the inner radius of the cup and radius of the femoral head. As the radial clearance increases, the contact area between the bearing surfaces decreases. Therefore, the optimal radial clearance provides polar bearing articulation and high conformity between bearing surfaces.

Further reading

Ashby M, Messler RW, Asthana R *et al* (2009). *Engineering Materials and Processes Desk Reference*. Oxford: Elsevier. 55–56.

Berrien LSJ (1999). Biotribology: Studies of the effect of biomechanical environments on the wear and damage of articular cartilage. PhD thesis. Virginia Polytechnic Institute and State University: USA.

Bucholz RW, Heckman JD, Court-Brown CM (eds) (2006). *Rockwood and Green's Fractures in Adults*. 6th edn. Philadelphia: Lippincott, Williams and Wilkins.

Callister, WD (2007). *Material Science and Engineering: An Introduction*. 7th edn. New York: Wiley.

Craig Jr RR (2011). *Mechanics of Materials*. 3rd edn. New York: John Wiley & Sons. 237–275.

Gayon J (2000). History of the concept of allometry. *Amer Zool*. 40: 748–758.

Johnson K (2001). *Physics for You*. London: Nelson Thornes.

Lee JY, Kim SY (2010). Alumina-on-polyethylene bearing surfaces in total hip arthroplasty. *Open Orthop J*. 4: 56–60.

Lucas GL, Cooke FW, Friis EA (1999). *A Primer of Biomechanics*. New York: Springer. 67–78.

Madihally SV (2010). *Principles of Biomedical Engineering*. Norwood: Artech House. 189–190.

Mansour JM (2008). Biomechanics of cartilage. In Oatis CA (ed): *Kinesiology: the Mechanics and Pathomechanics of Human Movement*. 2nd edn. 69–83.

Morgan EF, Bouxsein ML (2008). Biomechanics of bone and age-related fracture. In Bilezikian JP, Raisz LG, Martin TJ (eds): *Principles of Bone Biology*. 3rd edn. Vol 1. London: Elsevier. 29–52.

Neu CP, Komvopoulos K, Reddi AH (2008). The interface of functional biotribology and regenerative medicine in synovial joints. *Tissue Eng Part B Rev*. **14**(3): 235–247.

Nordin M, Frankel VH (2001). *Basic Biomechanics of the Musculoskeletal System*. 3rd edn. London: Lippincott, Williams and Wilkins.

Petit MA, Beck TJ, Kontulainen SA (2005). Examining the developing bone: What do we measure and how do we do it? *J Musculoskelet Neuronal Interact*. 5(3): 213–224.

Van der Meulen MCH, Jepsen KJ, Mikic B (2001). Understanding bone strength: size isn't everything. *Bone*. 29(2): 101–104.

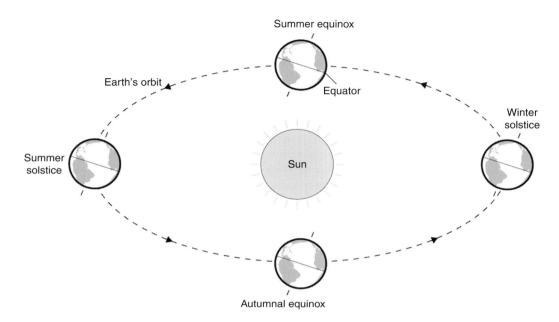

The Earth has an axis and orbit of motion. It rotates about its axis and orbits the Sun, with the orbital motion being superimposed on its spinning motion. The Earth's spinning axis is tilted 23.5° from the perpendicular to the plane of its orbit around the Sun. The rotation of the planet about its axis forms day and night. The tilt of the axis and the Earth's rotation around the Sun are responsible for the planet's seasons.

Similarly, in the musculoskeletal system, synovial joints also have axes and arcs of motion. The observable, main arc of motion of a joint is superimposed on top of smaller but essential motions in other planes. The understanding of orientation of normal axis and finer motions of a joint, and their significance to its overall functions is essential in joint reconstructive surgery.

Axes of the lower limbs

In the musculoskeletal system, an axis describes a plane within a structure, e.g. the axis of rotation of a joint and neutral axis in relation to bending and torsional loading of structures, or a plane of relative alignment of structures, e.g. axes of the lower limbs. It can sometimes be difficult to appreciate the three-dimensional orientation of the axes in the musculoskeletal system through descriptions and diagrams, and these are often better appreciated in a three-dimensional set-up, e.g. in computer/actual models or in a clinical/theatre setting.

The alignment of different bones and joints in the lower limbs is described by a number of axes. The comparison of these axes with each other and with different elements of the bones and joints can produce a constellation of angles and analyses. The alignment of the axes in the coronal plane is considered routinely, as lower limb deformities are more common in this plane. Therefore, the axes of the lower limb are discussed here in the coronal plane only, to simplify details and discuss important points. However, the alignment of these axes in the sagittal plane is also important and must also be considered where appropriate.

Anatomical axis

The anatomical axis describes the longitudinal anatomical alignment of the femur and tibia (i.e. the *bones*). This is conventionally represented by a line drawn down the centre of the diaphysis of each bone. The anatomical axes of the tibia and femur intersect at the knee at an average of 6° to each other.

Mechanical axis

The mechanical axis describes the alignment of the centres of the hip, knee and ankle *joints*. Conventionally, this is also described in terms of the bones, so that the mechanical axis of the femur is defined by a line connecting the centre of the femoral head to the medial tibial spine, and the mechanical axis of the tibia is defined by a line connecting the medial tibial spine with the centre of the ankle. The normal mechanical axis is not vertical, but is 3° valgus to the vertical, because the centre of the femoral head is in a valgus position with respect to the other joints.

Weight-bearing axis

The weight-bearing axis represents the path of load transmission to the ground relative to the lower limbs. It is represented by a line connecting the centre of the femoral head to the centre of the ankle.

The relationship between the axes

The anatomical axis of the femur is on average 6° valgus to its mechanical axis. The anatomical axis of the tibia is about 2–3° varus to its mechanical axis.

The normal mechanical axis overlaps the weight-bearing axis of the lower limbs; the mechanical axis is therefore commonly referred to as the weight-bearing axis.

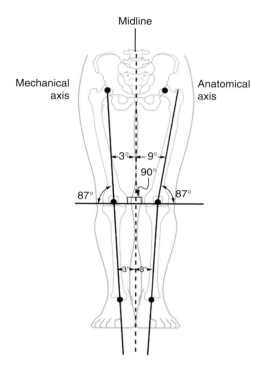

Fig. 6.1 The alignments of the anatomical and mechanical axes of the lower limbs. The anatomical axis of the femur is 6° valgus to its mechanical axis. The anatomical axis of the tibia is 2–3° varus to its mechanical axis, but the two tibial axes are considered to be identical for practical purposes, as the difference between them falls within the acceptable margin of error (<3°) in mechanical axis realignment during lower limb procedures, e.g. total knee replacement or deformity correction.

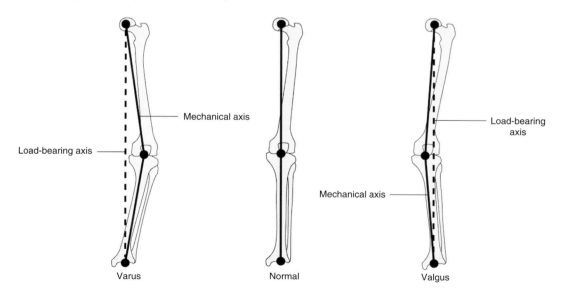

Fig. 6.2 The relationship between the mechanical and load-bearing axes of the lower limbs. The normal mechanical axis overlaps the load-bearing axis. In varus malalignment, the mechanical axis deviates lateral to the weight-bearing axis and in valgus malalignment it deviates medial to the load-bearing axis.

Hip joint reaction force I

Functional anatomy

The hip is a stable ball and socket joint, formed by the femoral head and pelvic acetabulum. The abductor muscles are the main stabilisers of the pelvis in the coronal plane. The total compressive force acting on the hip joint is the resultant of forces due to body weight, tension in the abductor muscles and any impact loads transmitted upwards through the body from the foot during everyday activities. A static analysis can be used to estimate the magnitude of hip joint reaction force under different circumstances.

Double-leg stance

The force acting on the hip joint during double-leg stance can be estimated from the proportional distribution of body weight. The legs comprise about 1/3 total body weight (TBW), so the weight of the upper body supported by the hips is approximately 2/3 TBW. Therefore, during a simple double-leg stance, each hip is subjected to a compressive force of about 1/3 TBW.

Assumptions
- During double-leg stance, abductor muscles are relaxed; any minimal tension (and therefore force) in abductor muscles is ignored.
- In a static situation, impact load transmitted from the ground is zero.

Single-leg stance

During a single-leg stance, the abductor muscles of the supporting leg contract to stabilise the pelvis. The hip joint acts as the axis of a class I lever and the pelvis acts as a rigid horizontal lever, supporting upper body weight on one side and abductor muscles force on the opposite side.

The proportional distribution of body weight means that the weight of the supported upper body is approximately 5/6 TBW. The abductor muscles generate a force to balance the moment produced by the upper body weight. According to Newton's third law, the joint reaction force must be equal and opposite to the sum of these two forces. The minimum hip joint reaction force is therefore estimated to be approximately 1.5 x TBW.

Assumptions
In addition to the general assumptions, the following specific assumptions are made in this analysis:
- The abductor muscles are the only active muscle group generating force, and there is no antagonistic muscle action.
- All forces are acting in a vertical direction. The line of action of the abductor muscles is actually 70° to the horizontal and therefore the abductor muscles actually produce a bit more force than estimated here.
- The pelvis is horizontal.
- In a static situation, impact load transmitted from the ground is zero.

Further exercise
The book cover shows a free-body force diagram showing forces acting on the right hip during a single-leg stance. Here it is assumed that the centre of gravity lies behind the public symphysis (this assumption is commonly made to simplify calculations). Could you calculate the abductor muscles force and hip joint reaction force in this example? Assume body weight = 600 N, A = 70 mm and B = 125 mm. (Answer is abductor muscles force = 1671 N and joint reaction force = 1671 N)

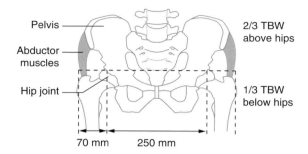

Fig. 6.3 The anatomical relationships between the hip joint, abductor muscles and the pelvis. Measurements provided are typical for an adult and are based on anthropometric data. During a double-leg stance, the centre of gravity of the supported upper body is in the midline and passes behind the pubic symphysis. (TBW= Total body weight.)

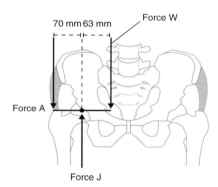

Fig. 6.4 Free-body force diagram of the pelvis showing the forces acting on the hip during a single-leg stance. The centre of gravity of the upper body shifts closer to the supporting hip to overlie the area of support, i.e. the foot, and is taken to be approximately halfway between the pubic symphysis and the centre of the hip joint. Each leg comprises 1/6 RV. The body weight below hips is 1/6 + 1/6 = 1/3 TBW. During single-leg stance weight of supported upper body is 2/3 + 1/6 = 5/6 TBW. (Force W = Weight of the upper body; Force A = Abductor muscles force; and, Force J = Joint reaction force.)

Calculations

Applying the conditions of equilibrium:

1. Sum of all moments is zero.

$\therefore$ Taking moments about the hip joint:
Total clockwise moments = Total anticlockwise moments
$$5/6 \text{ TBW} \times 0.063 = \text{Force } A \times 0.07$$
$$\text{Force } A = 3/4 \text{ TBW}$$

2. Sum of all forces is zero.

$\therefore$ Force J+($-$Force W)+($-$Force A) = 0
$$\text{Force } J - 5/6 \text{ TBW} - 3/4 \text{ TBW} = 0$$
$$\text{Force } J = 1\frac{1}{2} \text{ TBW}$$

The hip joint reaction force during single-leg stance. The joint reaction force is estimated to be about 1.5 × TBW.

Hip joint reaction force II

Single-leg stance with a cane support in the opposite hand

A cane support in the hand transmits force applied to it to the ground, and receives an equal and opposite ground reaction force, which it transmits back to the body. During a single-leg stance, when a cane is held in the opposite hand to the supporting hip, the class I lever system has an additional upwards-acting load, the ground reaction force, which has a longer lever arm than the supported upper body weight. This produces a moment in the same direction as the abductor muscles force. Therefore, the moments produced by abductor muscles force and ground reaction force both balance the moment produced by upper body weight, which reduces the force requirements of the abductor muscles. Therefore, the joint reaction force is reduced to about 1.3 x TBW during single-leg stance.

Assumptions

As discussed in the static analysis of hip joint reaction force during single-leg stance, plus:

- The weight of the cane is relatively small and is therefore ignored.

Single-leg stance with a 100 N load in the opposite hand

If a load is carried in the hands in normal everyday activities, this generates a downwards-acting force of weight. During a single-leg stance, when the load is held in the opposite hand to the supporting hip, the class I lever system has an additional downwards-acting force, the weight of the load, which has a longer lever arm than the upper body weight. This produces a moment in the same direction as the supported upper body weight. Therefore, the abductor muscles have to generate a force to balance two opposing moments, which significantly increases the force requirements of the abductor muscles. When a load of 100 N is carried in the opposite hand, the hip joint reaction force is estimated to be about 2.5 x TBW during single-leg stance.

Assumptions

As discussed in the hip joint reaction force analysis during single-leg stance.

Clinical implications

The hip joint reaction force during single-leg stance is more than the total body weight. The magnitude of the force is determined by the supported body weight, abductor muscles force and the ratio of their lever arms. The use of adjuncts can greatly influence the joint reaction force through their effect on these factors. The cane should be held in the opposite hand and any load, e.g. a shopping bag, should be carried in the same hand as the symptomatic hip, e.g. arthritic hip or during rehabilitation after a hip operation. In total hip replacement, 'medialising' the acetabular component increases the ratio of abductor muscles lever arm to the supported body weight lever arm, and therefore reduces the joint reaction force.

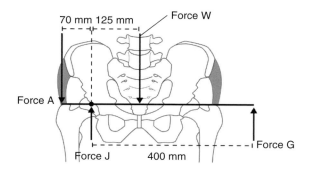

Fig. 6.5 Free-body force diagram of the pelvis showing the forces acting on the hip during a single-leg stance with a cane support in the opposite hand. The cane support provides stability through an additional point of contact with the ground, and improves the body's centre of gravity to a wider, stable range. Therefore, the centre of gravity of the supported upper body lies behind the pubic symphysis (as in the double-leg stance). The ground reaction force is limited by the force that can be applied to the cane by the upper limb, which in an adult is typically about 100 N (or 1/7 TBW), taken to act at 400 mm from the supporting hip. (Force W = Weight of the upper body; Force A = Abductor muscles force; Force J = Joint reaction force; and Force G = Ground reaction force acting on the cane.)

Calculations

Applying the conditions of equilibrium:

1. Sum of all moments is zero.

∴ Taking moments about the hip joint:

Total clockwise moments = Total anticlockwise moments

$$5/6 \text{ TBW} \times 0.125 = (\text{Force } A \times 0.07) + (1/7 \text{ TBW} \times 0.4)$$
$$\text{Force } A = 2/3 \text{ TBW}$$

2. Sum of all forces is zero.

∴ Force J + Force G + (−Force W) + (−Force A) = 0

Force J − 1/7 TBW − 5/6 TBW − 2/3 TBW = 0

$$\therefore \text{Force } J = 1\frac{1}{3} \text{ TBW}$$

The hip joint reaction force during single-leg stance with cane support in the opposite hand. The joint reaction force is about 1.3 × TBW.

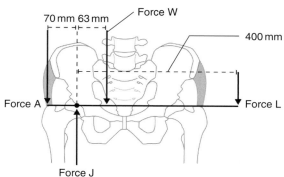

Fig. 6.6 Free-body force diagram of the pelvis showing the forces acting on the hip during a single-leg stance with a 100 N load in the opposite hand. The centre of gravity of the supported upper body weight shifts closer to the supporting hip as in the simple single-leg stance. In an adult, a 100 N load is 1/7 TBW and is taken to act at 400 mm from the supporting hip. (L = Weight of the load.)

Calculations

Applying the conditions of equilibrium

1. Sum of all moments is zero.

∴ Taking moments about the hip joint :

Total clockwise moments = Total anticlockwise moments

$$(5/6 \text{ TBW} \times 0.063) + (1/7 \text{ TBW} \times 0.4) = (\text{Force } A \times 0.07)$$
$$\text{Force } A = 1\frac{1}{2} \text{ TBW}$$

2. Sum of all forces is zero.

∴ Force J + (−Force W) + (−Force A) + (−Force L) = 0

Force J − 5/6 TBW − $1\frac{1}{2}$ TBW − 1/7 TBW = 0

$$\text{Force } J = 2\frac{1}{2} \text{ TBW}$$

The hip joint reaction force during single-leg stance with a 100 N load in the opposite hand. The joint reaction force is about 2½ x TBW.

Total hip replacement (THR): cemented fixation

Fixation of total hip replacement implants to bones with cement provides immediate stability to the construct. Cement functions as grout, and not as an adhesive, to provide a mechanical interlock between implant and bone. As cement does not stimulate new bone formation and there is no renewal of bonding at the cement–bone interface, the quality of cemented fixation degrades with time.

Femoral stem implant design

There are two basic designs of cemented fixation femoral stem implant, which interact with cement differently to achieve durable stability.

Composite beam

This type of stem has a small protrusion, a collar, at the level of the femoral calcar; a pre-coated, roughened fixation surface; and a cylindrical profile throughout its length. These features optimise the stem for a strong bond with cement. The proximal collar prevents distal sinkage of the stem, and the rough fixation surface ensures maximum bonding between stem and cement.

The proximal collar also increases the load transferred from stem to the femoral calcar, aiming to replicate natural load transmission in the proximal femur. The extensive bonding between stem and cement maintains the stem in its position without any slip within the cement mantle; therefore, it is considered a 'sit up and stay' prosthesis. The firm fixation achieved does not accommodate creep within the cement mantle. The load is transferred to the femur by shear stress at the bone–cement interface. Due to all these characteristics, the stem is described as having a 'shape closed' design.

Taper slip

This type of stem is collarless; has a highly polished fixation surface; and has a tapered profile from proximal to distal. These features prevent the stem from bonding with cement. The stem therefore settles in cement, re-engaging its taper, and so the fixation becomes progressively more stable; therefore it is considered a 'slip and slide' prosthesis. The re-engagement of the taper converts shear stress at the interface into radial compression of cement. The load is therefore transferred to the femur by compressive stress at the bone–cement interface. As the stem is mobile, it can accommodate creep within the cement mantle. Due to all these characteristics, the stem is described as having a 'force closed' design.

The effect of surface finish

The polished surface finish is an essential feature of the taper slip stem. The stem has been trialled with a matte surface finish (as polishing is a labour-intensive and expensive process), and was found to have a significantly high failure rate (revision rate 10% at 10 years, compared with 2.5% at 10 years for a polished surface finish). The matte surface finish leads to the stem bonding with cement, although its features are not suited for this. The matte taper slip stem is unable to settle in cement and convert the shear forces to compressive forces and therefore has a higher failure rate.

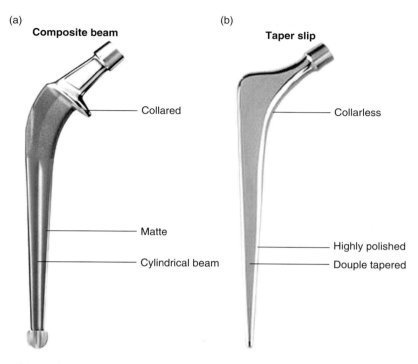

Fig. 6.7 Comparison of design features of the two types of cemented fixation femoral stem implant. (a) The composite beam stem is also referred to as the 'Charnley' stem, as it was developed by Charnley and Harris in the 1950s. (b) The taper slip stem is also referred to as the 'Exeter' stem, as it was developed in Exeter by Ling and Lee in the 1970s. (Image (a) is reproduced with permission of Smith & Nephew. Image (b) is reprinted from Choy GG *et al*. (2013) Exeter short stems compared with standard length Exeter stems: experience from the Australian Orthopaedic Association National Joint Replacement Registry. *J Arthroplasty*. 28(1): 103–109. Copyright (2013) with permission from Elsevier.)

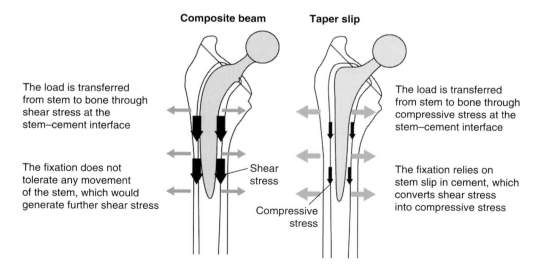

Fig. 6.8 Comparison of load transfer between the two types of cemented fixation femoral stem implant. The stem–bone construct is a composite, and is subjected to the same loads as the natural hip. The implant is much stiffer than bone and therefore accepts more load, which it then transfers to the bone.

Total hip replacement: cementless fixation

Total hip replacements with cementless fixation are being increasingly used in younger patients to preserve bone stock and avoid problems associated with cemented fixation. The 'press fit' placement of implant in the bone cavity achieves initial stability, and implant osteo-integration provides long-term stability. Cementless fixation is therefore a biological fixation, which is dynamic because of bone turnover and therefore the quality of fixation is maintained with time.

Femoral stem implant design

A cementless fixation femoral stem has a porous and/or a biologically active fixation surface. A biologically active interface is formed by a textured surface finish or coating the implant with a biologically active material. A textured surface is very finely rough, e.g. like sandpaper, and is produced by grit-blasting the stem. The commonly used bioactive materials for application to the implants are commercially pure titanium or ceramics, i.e. hydroxyapatite. The biological fixation of implant is achieved by bone ingrowth into the porous surface or ongrowth to the biologically active surface. During the bonding process, new bone can tolerate only small movements of the stem (up to 28 μm), and does not form if there is excessive motion (more than 150 μm); in which case a layer of connective tissue forms between the stem and bone.

The early cementless fixation femoral stems (e.g. the 'fully' porous coated stems) were cylindrical and prepared up to distal diaphyseal section to biologically bond with the bone. The extensive bonding achieved in the femoral diaphysis produced problems of stress shielding of proximal femur (i.e. stress protection osteopenia), thigh pain and difficulty removing the implant at revision. Therefore, most uncemented femoral stems are now tapered and prepared for osteo-integration in the proximal part only. Distal fixation stems are mainly used in revision surgery, e.g. for periprosthetic fractures. These revision stems have different cross-section designs and may also have the option of interlocking screw fixation.

Cemented fixation vs cementless fixation

Clinical studies comparing the results of total hip replacements with cemented and cementless fixations show that cemented fixation has better overall long-term results (i.e. lower revision rates), but cementless fixation appears to have advantages in certain situations. Cementless fixation has potentially better resistance to aseptic loosening in the younger patients, and the long-term outcome of total hip replacements with cementless fixation does not appear to be affected by varus or valgus mal-alignment of the femoral stem.

Cementless fixation is associated with a higher rate of intra-operative fractures. The common mechanism of intra-operative fractures is generation of excessive hoop stresses during preparation of bone and insertion of prosthesis. The impaction of prosthesis to achieve press fit fixation with the bone in cementless fixation leads to a higher occurrence of excessive hoop stresses generation; whereas cemented fixation does not require such compact fixation (Tables 6.1 and 6.2).

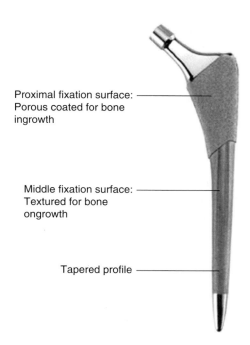

Proximal fixation surface:
Porous coated for bone
ingrowth

Middle fixation surface:
Textured for bone
ongrowth

Tapered profile

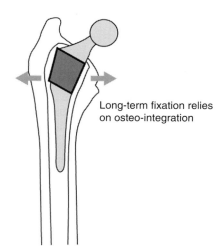

Long-term fixation relies
on osteo-integration

Fig. 6.9 Design features of a typical cementless fixation femoral stem implant. (Image is reproduced with permission of Smith & Nephew.)

Fig. 6.10 Load transfer from stem to bone in cementless fixation femoral stem. The stem is designed to transfer load mainly at the metaphyseal section as shear stress at the implant–bone interface.

Table 6.1. **Hybrid fixation**

Aseptic loosening of the acetabular component is commonly the limiting factor to the long-term survivorship of cemented total hip replacement. Therefore, sometimes hybrid fixation is used so that there is cementless fixation of the acetabular component and cemented fixation of the femoral component.

Cementless fixation acetabular component is formed of a metal cup with a separate inlay of the bearing surface. The component is press fixed to the acetabulum. The fixation surface is bioactive for bonding with the bone, but the component can also be further secured with screws.

A 'reverse hybrid' fixation may also be used which consists of a cemented acetabular (usually polyethylene) component and a cementless fixation femoral stem.

Table 6.2. **Percentage of primary total hip replacements (THR) performed in the UK over a 10-year period (Data taken from National Joint Registry report 2014)**

Fixation type	Year										
	2003	2004	2005	2006	2007	2008	2009	2010	2011	2012	2013
Cemented fixation	60.5	54.1	48.6	42.8	39.7	34.3	31.9	31.4	38.3	32.9	33.2
Cementless fixation	16.8	21.4	25.6	30.1	33.3	39.4	43.2	45.8	44.9	44.9	42.5
Hybrid	12.3	13.3	14.1	15.2	15.0	15.1	15.8	16.2	17.2	17.7	20.2
Reverse hybrid	0.6	0.9	1.1	1.2	1.7	2.5	2.7	2.8	3.1	3.1	3.0
Resurfacing	9.8	10.2	10.7	10.8	10.2	8.8	6.5	3.8	2.5	1.4	1.1
Actual number of THR performed	14 413	27 993	40 150	47 523	60 460	66 707	67 547	69 891	72 835	76 607	76 274

Can you spot the general trends?

Total hip replacement: design and alignment of components

The main biomechanical goals of total hip replacement are to: restore the centre of rotation of the joint; maintain mechanical axis of the lower limb; preserve leg length; and achieve correct soft tissue balance. The design and alignment of components are key factors in determining the performance of the replacement hip joint. It is important to undertake pre-operative planning, which helps to establish the correct size, design and alignment of components.

Design

In the femoral component, neck length and off-set determine the neck-shaft angle and abductor muscles lever arm. Correct restoration of these variables is important for proper soft tissue balancing of the hip. A change in neck length has a greater effect on leg length than the abductors muscles lever arm, whereas a change in off-set affects the abductor muscles lever arm more than leg length. Therefore, to optimise the abductor muscles lever arm, it is better to increase the off-set than the neck of the implant.

A polyethylene acetabular cup can be used with or without a 20° elevation 'posterior lip augmentation device'. The elevated posterior lip reduces the risk of total hip replacement dislocation; however, it also decreases the primary arc of motion. Dislocations can still occur, especially in very active persons, due to femoral neck impingement on the prominent acetabular cup. Other 'constrained' liners are also available to further enclose the femoral head, which are used most commonly in revision surgery for instability.

Alignment

Component alignment is a function of its position within the bone cavity and orientation with respect to the body. The femoral stem should be positioned valgus in the coronal plane and parallel in the sagittal plane with respect to the bone cortices; varus and 'back to front' placement must be avoided, especially in cemented fixation, as the normal eccentric loading produces bending forces that are pushing the stem in these directions.

Normally, the optimum position of the acetabular cup is 'medialised' within the acetabulum. This achieves the best combination of bone/cup coverage for fixation interface and cup/femoral head coverage to reduce contact stresses at the bearing interface. Medialising the acetabular cup also reduces joint reaction force, by increasing the lever arm of the abductor muscles and decreasing the lever arm of body weight. The position of the acetabular cup within the acetabulum is decided at the time of the operation.

The safe zone of orientation of components to minimise the risk of impingement and dislocation is as follows:

- *Femoral stem*:   Axial plane (anteversion angle): 0°–20°
- *Acetabular cup*:   Coronal plane (theta angle): 40° +/− 10°
  Sagittal plane (anteversion angle): 15° +/− 10°.

Practically, the acetabular cup normally is aligned with the transverse acetabular ligament during the operation. This automatically ensures the correct orientation of the acetabular component, and fine adjustments can then be made as required.

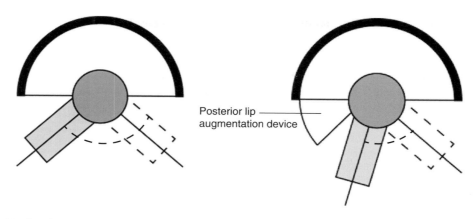

Posterior lip augmentation device

Fig. 6.11 A 20° elevation posterior lip augmentation device provides a greater femoral head cover and helps to reduce dislocations, but also reduces the primary arc of motion.

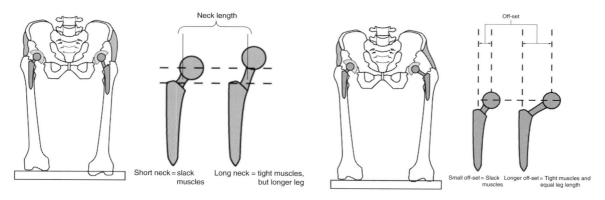

Fig. 6.12 The effect of increasing the neck length and off-set of femoral component on leg length and abductor muscles tensioning. The off-set required in the femoral component is determined by taking measurements on the pre-operative radiographs.

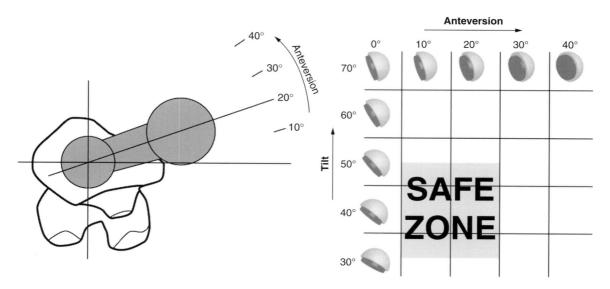

Fig. 6.13 The safe zone of orientation of femoral and acetabular components.

Total hip replacement: femoral head size

The femoral head diameter is an important determinant of the range of motion, stability and wear properties of the replacement joint. Range of motion and stability are related and are a function of the head–neck ratio. The head–neck ratio increases with a larger diameter femoral head or with a tapered (narrower) neck. A greater head–neck ratio permits a wider primary arc of motion before impingement of components. Therefore, a greater head–neck ratio offers better range of motion and stability. In addition, a larger diameter femoral head also requires a greater displacement for dislocation, i.e. 'jump distance', and therefore offers further stability.

Wear of the bearing surfaces of total hip replacement can be measured in two ways:

- *Linear wear.* The thickness of the acetabular cup decreases as it wears with use. Linear wear is the change in the thickness of the acetabular cup with time, and is measured as follows:

    Linear wear [mm] = Original thickness of acetabular cup [mm] – New shortest thickness of acetabular cup [mm], as measured on a plain AP radiograph.

- *Volumetric wear.* This describes the actual volume of wear of the acetabular component. Volumetric wear is related to linear wear with this simple geometry-based equation:

    Volumetric wear [mm^3] = π x (radius of femoral head [mm])^2 x linear wear [mm]

    Therefore, a larger diameter femoral head produces more volumetric wear for the same linear wear.

Wear between different femoral head sizes and bearing combinations

Volumetric wear is proportional to the frictional torque of the replacement joint. The formula for frictional torque is:

$$\text{Frictional torque [N m]} = \text{Friction [N]} \times \text{Distance from centre of rotation [m]}$$
$$\therefore \text{Frictional torque [N m]} = \mu \times \text{Joint load [N]} \times \text{Radius of femoral head [m]}$$

See pages 82–83 for further explanation.

Therefore, an increase in femoral head size increases frictional torque and related volumetric wear. However, different bearing materials have different coefficients of friction and therefore produce different amounts of wear for the same femoral head size.

Example

Metal head on polyethylene acetabular cup is the most commonly used bearing combination. In the past, a 28 mm diameter femoral head was considered to provide the optimum balance between stability and wear. Now, other bearing materials with better wear properties are used to develop larger diameter femoral heads.

The primary arcs of motion for a 28 mm and a 36 mm diameter femoral head are 123° and 136°, respectively. In metal on polyethylene bearing combination, this increase in femoral head size increases frictional torque by 1.29 times and volumetric wear by 2.6 times. The coefficient of friction of ceramic on ceramic bearing combination is 1.33 times less than metal on polyethylene bearing combination. Therefore, for the same increase in femoral head size, it experiences practically no increase in frictional torque, and the increase in volumetric wear is 100 times less.

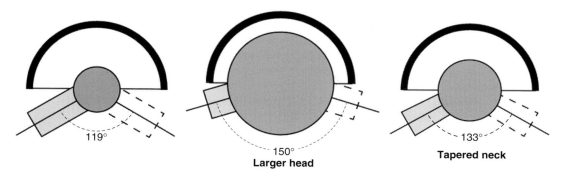

Fig. 6.14 The effect of head–neck ratio on primary arc of motion. A greater head–neck ratio permits a wider primary arc of motion before impingement of components. Note that the outer diameter of the acetabular cup remains the same.

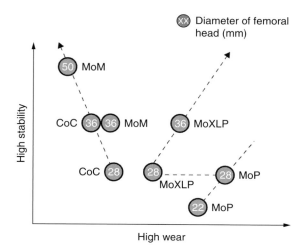

Fig. 6.15 A larger diameter femoral head requires a bigger jump distance before dislocation. It also reduces the empty space around the acetabular component into which it can dislocate. These factors make it more difficult to dislocate a larger size femoral head.

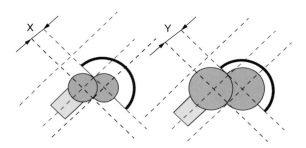

Fig. 6.16 The relationship of wear and stability with femoral head size and bearing combinations. A larger diameter femoral head provides more stability, but in a metal on polyethylene (MoPE) bearing combination produces excessive wear that leads to osteolysis and implant loosening. Other bearing combinations, i.e. metal on highly cross-linked polyethylene (MoXLPE), metal on metal (MoM) and ceramic on ceramic (CoC), have much lower coefficients of friction and permit the use of larger diameter femoral head with less wear. In fact, wear in MoM and CoC combinations decreases with an increase in femoral head diameter, because fluid film lubrication takes effect as the femoral head diameter increases (see pages 92–93).

Total hip replacement: bearing surfaces

Two of the main reasons for revising a total hip replacement are aseptic loosening and instability, i.e. dislocations. Different combinations of bearing surfaces present various solutions to these problems, but also have their own limitations. The governing factors that connect different bearing surfaces combinations to aseptic loosening and instability are as follows:

(a) *Osteolysis.* This is the main cause of aseptic loosening. Wear particles from mainly the acetabular cup produce a biological reaction that leads to osteolysis and implant loosening.

(b) *Femoral head diameter.* Although a larger diameter femoral head offers a greater range of motion and is more stable, it also leads to increased wear.

Metal on polyethylene

Metal femoral head on polyethylene acetabular cup is the most commonly used bearing combination, and has a well-established clinical track record. Femoral heads of 22 mm and 28 mm diameter have been used traditionally, as a bigger femoral head increases polyethylene wear rate. The newer 'highly cross-linked' polyethylene is harder and produces about 60% less wear, and is encouraging the use of larger diameter femoral heads. This is the only combination where a posterior lip augmentation device can be applied to the acetabular cup to reduce the risk of dislocation.

Metal on metal

In this combination, femoral head and acetabular cup are both made of metal. As metals are hard materials, this is a described as a 'hard on hard' bearing combination. In addition, metals can be polished to reduce surface roughness, which further reduces wear. Therefore, larger size ($\geq$36 mm) femoral heads can be used, as even the increased wear rate is still a magnitude less than in metal on polyethylene combination. Metal on metal combination can also retain fluid between the bearing surfaces and therefore can achieve fluid film lubrication, which further minimises wear.

Ceramic on ceramic

In ceramic on ceramic bearing combination, the femoral head and acetabular cup are both made from ceramic material. As ceramics are harder than metals, these can be highly polished. Ceramic on ceramic combination is therefore very hard and smooth. Ceramics are also hydrophilic and very 'wettable', which means that ceramic bearing surfaces can more easily achieve fluid film lubrication. Therefore, ceramic on ceramic bearings have the lowest clinical wear rate of any bearing combination.

Other bearing combinations

Oxinium^{TM} is a relatively new bearing surface that consists of a metal femoral head with a ceramic surface coating, for use with a ceramic acetabular cup. It combines the benefits of both materials: metal femoral head cannot fracture and the ceramic surface has a very low wear rate with no issues regarding the accumulation of metal ions. It is, however, very expensive, and there are limited long-term clinical data (Table 6.3).

Table 6.3. A summary of main advantages and disadvantages of different bearing combinations

	Advantages	Disadvantages
Metal on polyethylene	Predictable performance and failure mechanisms. Local biological effects only. Forgiving materials: performance is not affected in a wide range of alignment of implants. Polyethylene acetabular cup available: • in a large range of sizes • with posterior lip augmentation device, and other constraint designs • in highly cross-linked composition. Revision options are not limited. Relatively cheap.	Osteolysis and aseptic loosening: • does not support fluid film lubrication • high wear rates with larger femoral head sizes. Highly cross-linked polyethylene is: • brittle, and susceptible to fracture • less forgiving of implant mal-alignment.
Metal on metal	Virtually no risk of fracture (although the components are still prone to scratches). Low wear rate. 'Hip resurfacing' implants are only available in metal on metal combination, as only this combination can endure the design in the long term. Long history of use.	Effects of metal ions wear particles: • immunological effects: Avascular lymphocytic vascular associated lesions (ALVAL) and Lymphocyte dominated immunological answer (LYDIA). • chromosomal aberrations. • toxicity. • pseudotumours. • potentially carcinogenic. Requires long-term patient follow-up to monitor for issues relating to metal ions. Absolute contraindications: • renal failure (as metals ions accumulate in kidneys) • women of child-bearing age (unknown effect of metal ions on the foetus).
Ceramic on ceramic	Lowest wear rate. Biological inert wear particles, therefore low inflammatory reaction and osteolysis, and no issues of ion toxicity.	Performance very sensitive to implant alignment; susceptible to catastrophic fracture if components slightly out of alignment. Very fine wear debris, which is difficult to remove at revision surgery, therefore revision options often restricted to the same combination. Can sometimes produce audible noise when walking, e.g. squeaking or clicking. More expensive than other bearing options.

Knee: functional anatomy I

The knee is the largest and most complex joint in the body. It is an articulation among the distal femur, proximal tibia and patella, surrounded by a soft tissue envelope of capsule, ligaments, tendons and muscles. The specific anatomical features and interactions of these structures determine the stability and movements of the knee joint.

Geometry and alignment of the bones

Tibiofemoral joint

The medial tibial plateau is larger than the lateral tibial plateau. It also has a concave depression whereas the lateral tibial plateau has a convex surface. Both plateaux have a posterior tilt of about 7°, but the joint surface tilt is minimised to 3° by the menisci. The plateaux also have a 3° varus tilt, i.e. the joint surface is slopped medially.

On the femoral side, the medial condyle is larger, more curved and extends more distally than the lateral condyle.

This asymmetry between the medial and lateral compartments of the knee determines the relative mobility of each compartment. The concave medial tibial plateau offers more constraint and the convex lateral tibial plateau offers less constraint to the movements of their respective femoral condyles. The posterior and varus tilts of the tibial plateaux have implication for the alignment of bone cuts for total knee replacement.

Patellofemoral joint

The patella is a sesamoid bone that articulates with the femur only. It has two articular facets: the lateral facet is slightly larger than the medial facet. The quadriceps tendon and patellar tendon insert at the anterior aspect of the patella, and its thickness increases the extension lever arm of the quadriceps muscle. This effect is maximum in full knee extension and reduces with knee flexion, when the patella sinks into the intercondylar groove. Due to the mechanical advantage provided by the patella, the quadriceps needs to generate about 20%–30% less force for a certain extension torque. The medial and lateral facets of the patella also increase the surface area over which the compressive stress is applied to the femur. The patella also protects the tibiofemoral joint from direct trauma.

The Q-angle (quadriceps angle) describes patella alignment. It is formed by lines connecting the centre of patella with the anterior superior iliac spine proximally and the centre of tibial tubercle distally. The normal Q-angle range is 10°–14° for males and 15°–17° for females; the Q-angle is greater in females, as they generally have a wider pelvic girdle. The greater the Q-angle, the greater the lateral force on the patella, and a Q-angle more than 20° is a risk factor for patella subluxation and patellofemoral joint pain. The restoration of the normal Q-angle is important in total knee replacement for normal patella tracking.

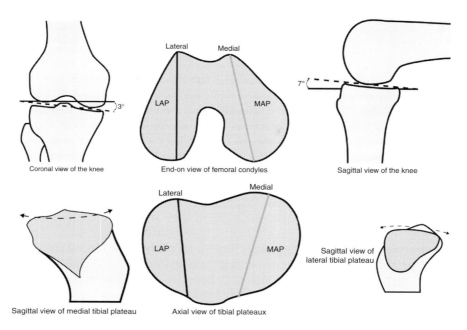

Fig. 7.1 Geometry of articular surfaces of femoral condyles and tibial plateaux. (LAP = Lateral anteroposterior diameter; MAP = Medial anteroposterior diameter.)

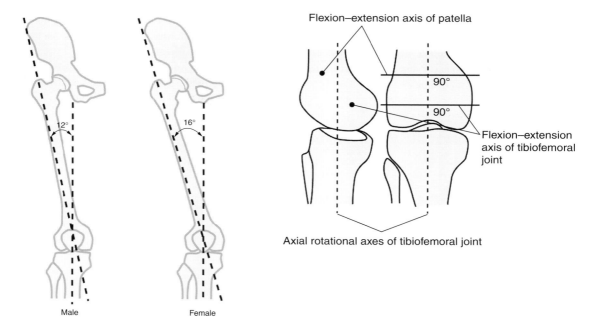

Fig. 7.2 The Q-angle is formed by lines connecting the centre of patella with the anterior superior iliac spine proximally and the centre of tibial tubercle distally. The Q-angle is greater in females because they generally have a wider pelvic girdle. The greater the Q-angle, the greater the lateral force on the patella.

Fig. 7.3 There are three axes of the knee joint: flexion–extension and axial rotational axes of tibiofemoral joint and flexion–extension axis of the patella. The flexion–extension axis of the tibiofemoral joint is also referred to as the transepicondylar axis or the surgical epicondylar axis. It is defined by a line that connects the lateral epicondylar prominence to the medial epicondylar sulcus. There is a parallel and orthogonal relationship between the axes.

113

Knee: functional anatomy II

Soft tissues of the knee

The cruciate ligaments

The anterior and posterior cruciate ligaments are the primary restraint to anterior and posterior translation of tibia, respectively. The cruciate ligaments function in a special configuration, which in mechanical terms is known as the 'four-bar linkage mechanism'. In this model, the cruciate ligaments form the two crossed bars and the bones effectively form the other two bars. As the knee joint flexes and extends, the cruciate ligaments are able to pivot about their insertion points. The length of the four bars remains constant, but the angle between them changes during joint motion. In addition, the centre of rotation of this four-bar linkage hinge is at the crossover point of the cruciate ligaments, which also changes with knee position. The cruciate ligaments are not rigid and experience some change in length, which allows internal–external rotation of the joint. The ligaments set-up is therefore described as 'modified' (as opposed to rigid) four-bar linkage mechanism.

The menisci

The medial and lateral menisci increase the congruency between the tibial and the femoral articular surfaces. The medial meniscus is attached to the medial joint capsule, and the lateral meniscus is attached to the femur by the meniscofemoral ligament. Therefore, during knee flexion, the lateral meniscus translates posteriorly much more than the medial meniscus. The menisci contribute to stability and facilitate movements of the knee joint.

The menisci also help to distribute knee joint load over maximum contact area. The compressive load from the femur is transmitted to the 'menisco-tibial' interface, with the menisci carrying approximately 70% of the load across the knee joint. The removal of menisci results in load transmitted through a limited, central contact area, which leads to a three- to five-fold increase in the stress applied to the articular surfaces. The menisci therefore protect the articular surfaces from excessive stresses.

A further function of the menisci is as 'shock absorbers' of the knee joint. They reduce the actual load transmitted across the knee joint by dissipating axial stress through generation of hoop stresses. The menisci deform elastically when loaded, and experience radial and circumferential stresses. The circumferential, or hoop, stresses are in a different plane to joint loading planes, which reduces the stress transmitted across the menisci.

The menisci are viscoelastic and also display hysteresis, which is the ability to absorb energy when subjected to repeated loading and unloading cycles. This energy is dissipated in changing the shape of the menisci during loading and unloading.

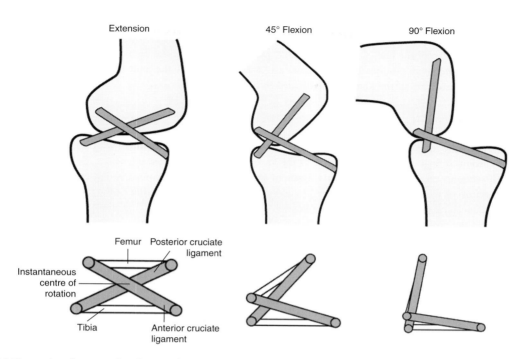

Fig. 7.4 The cruciate ligaments function as a four-bar linkage hinge to stabilise the joint whilst permitting motion.

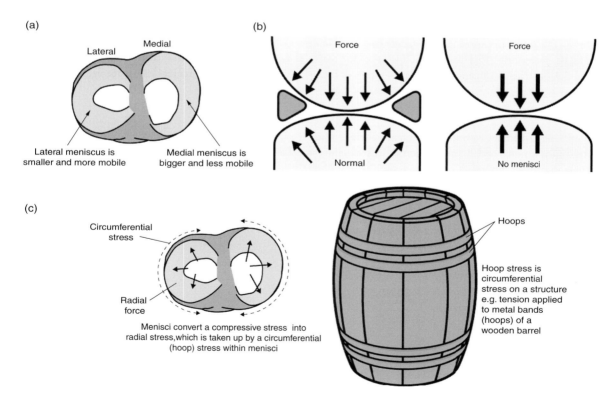

Fig. 7.5 The biomechanical functions of the menisci are to (a) stabilise the articulating surfaces and facilitate joint motion; (b) distribute joint load over maximum contact area; and (c) act as shock absorbers by generating hoop stresses.

Knee: flexion–extension arc

The main arc of motion of the knee joint is flexion and extension in the sagittal plane. However, the knee is not a simple hinge joint and small motions in other planes are essential to enable the joint to flex and extend.

The flexion–extension arc of the knee can be divided into three ranges.

Screw home arc

−5° to 10°: This is the range where the knee is 'locked'. The femur is in neural alignment with the tibia when the knee is at 10° of flexion. It begins to internally rotate as the knee extends. In full knee extension: the femur is internally rotated with reference to the tibia; the cruciate ligament four-bar linkage mechanism is tightened; and the joint is locked. The centre of weight of the upper body lies anterior to the centre of rotation of the joint, and the resultant moment is balanced by passive resistance of the posterior capsule and ligaments. This allows the quadriceps to stop contracting and the position is maintained passively with little energy expenditure.

The knee is 'unlocked' by the action of the popliteus located at the posterolateral corner of the knee, and the femur begins to externally rotate as knee flexion is initiated.

Functional arc

10° to 120°: This range is associated with further external rotation of the femur. This is because, as the knee flexes, the smaller lateral femoral condyle also begins to slide posteriorly, whereas the larger medial femoral condyle maintains its relative position on the tibia, which therefore has the overall effect of externally rotating the femur. This is considered an 'active' range, because the ligaments and muscles are controlling the rate of motion.

Deep flexion arc

120° to 145°/160°: In this range, the femur continues to externally rotate and, in addition, both femoral condyles translate posteriorly. This 'rollback and slide' of the femur allows the femoral condyles to clear the tibia to achieve deep flexion. This is considered a 'passive' range, as it can only be achieved with manual assistance or by squatting.

Patellofemoral contact zones

The patella articulates with the lateral femoral ridge when the knee is in full extension, and slides into the intercondylar notch at full knee flexion. This sliding of patella along the femur brings specific zones of femur and patella in contact during different ranges of the flexion–extension arc. The contact area becomes more proximal on the patella and more distal on the femur with increasing knee flexion. The size of the patellofemoral contact area also increases with knee flexion, i.e. with increased force of the quadriceps. When the knee is at 30° of flexion, patellar contact area is about 2 cm^2, and when it is at 90° of flexion, the contact area triples to about 6 cm^2. This maintains stress at the patellofemoral joint at a relatively constant level despite an increase in quadriceps force with increasing knee flexion (Table 7.1).

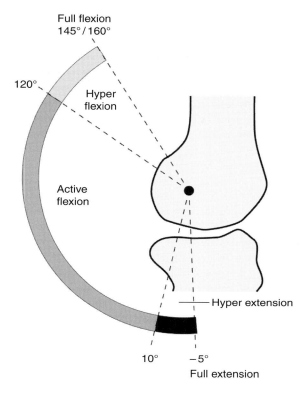

Fig. 7.6 The flexion–extension arc of the knee can be divided into three ranges, which are associated with specific motions of the femur over the tibia.

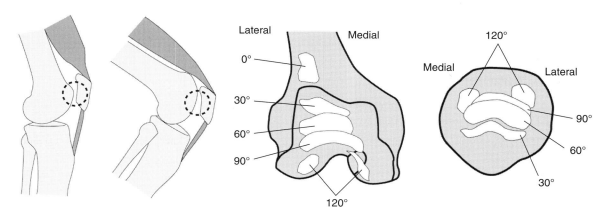

Fig. 7.7 Patellofemoral contact zones during the flexion–extension arc. The contact area becomes more proximal on the patella and more distal on the femur with increasing knee flexion.

Table 7.1 **A note on the flexion–extension arc**

The flexion–extension arc of the knee is described here in terms of the alignment of the femur with respect to the tibia with increasing knee flexion. It can also be described in terms of the alignment of tibia with respect to femur and/or in terms of increasing knee extension. The description of the relative motion between the bones will change accordingly in these cases.

Knee joint reaction force

Static analysis can be used to estimate the compressive forces acting on tibiofemoral and patellofemoral joints. These forces increase with knee flexion angle, and also depend on whether the leg is in the stance or swing phase of the gait cycle. The stance phase is further divided into double-leg and single-leg support periods. The knee joint reaction forces are greatest at maximum knee flexion during the single-leg stance period of the gait cycle. However, maximum knee flexion during the single-leg stance period varies according to the activity undertaken, e.g. it is approximately 20° walking on flat surface, 60° ascending stairs and 85° descending stairs (Table 7.2). As a result, the joint reaction forces produced in the knee compartments are very variable, and any analysis must take into account the exact loading conditions.

Tibiofemoral joint reaction force

During a simple double- or single-leg stance: the knee is in full extension; there is no resultant moment due to the supported upper body weight; and the quadriceps muscles are not contracting. The tibiofemoral joint reaction force is roughly equal to the supported upper body weight. The weight of the leg below the knee is about 5% of total body weight and can be ignored; therefore, each tibiofemoral joint is subjected to a compressive force equivalent to one-half of total body weight during double-leg stance and total body weight during single-leg stance.

The tibiofemoral joint reaction force increases sharply with knee flexion. It is the resultant vector of the ground reaction force and quadriceps force. A commonly used example to illustrate the peak forces produced in the tibiofemoral joint is during ascending stairs. The typical height of a step of stairs is 20 cm, which requires about 60° of knee flexion during the single-leg stance period of the gait cycle. The static analysis shows that tibiofemoral joint reaction force is about five times total body weight.

Assumptions

In addition to the general assumptions, the following specific assumptions are applied to this static analysis:

- The quadriceps provides all of the force to extend the knee and exerts a tensile force through the patella tendon.
- The ground reaction force is equal and opposite to total body weight, and acts below the centre of weight of the body.
- The following physical measurements are based on anthropometric data:
  - Moment arm of patella tendon at 60° of knee flexion is 45 mm.
  - Moment arm of ground reaction force at 60° of knee flexion is 180 mm.

Patellofemoral joint reaction force

The compressive force in the patellofemoral joint is the resultant vector of the patella tendon and quadriceps tendon forces, and also increases with knee flexion. At 60° of knee flexion during single-leg stance in ascending stairs, the patellofemoral joint reaction force is estimated to be about four times total body weight.

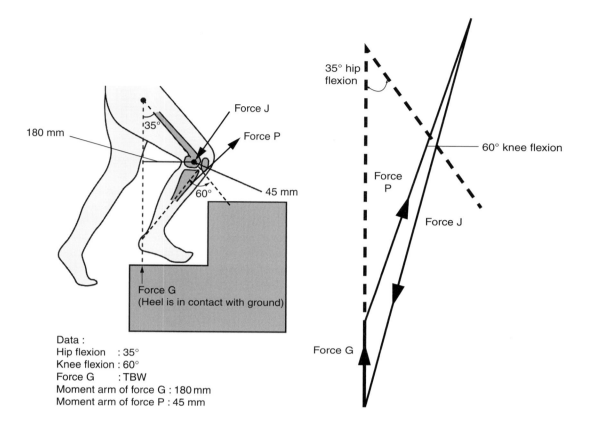

Data :
Hip flexion : 35°
Knee flexion : 60°
Force G : TBW
Moment arm of force G : 180 mm
Moment arm of force P : 45 mm

Fig. 7.8 Free-body force diagram of the knee joint during ascending stairs at the instance of opposite foot toe-off. The tibiofemoral joint is acting as a class I lever. The actual degree of knee flexion required to ascend stairs is determined by the height of the step as well as the height of the person. For a standard 20 cm rise and 30 cm run step, on average 60° of knee flexion is required. This is associated with approximately 35° of hip flexion.

Moment arm of ground reaction force is usually four times the moment arm of patella tendon at *any* degree of knee flexion. (Force G = Ground reaction force; Force P = Patella tendon force; and Force J = Joint reaction force.)

Calculations

Applying the conditions of equilibrium:

1. Sum of all moments is zero.

∴ Taking moments about the knee joint:
Total clockwise moments = Total anticlockwise moments
$$TBW \times 0.18 = P \times 0.045$$
$$P = 4TBW$$

2. Sum of all forces is zero.

∴ A graphical method can be used to determine Force J.
Scale: 10 mm = 1TBW

Tibiofemoral joint reaction force during ascending stairs. The joint reaction force is about five times total body weight (TBW).

Total knee replacement (TKR): design of components I

Total knee replacement involves resurfacing the femoral condyles and tibial surfaces with or without resurfacing the patella. Modern total knee replacement implants have the following design features in common:

- The metal-based femoral component has two symmetrical runners that are bridged at the anterior aspect to form an articular surface for the patella.
- The polyethylene tibial insert has two concave articular surfaces.
- The polyethylene patellar component is circular and has a convex articular surface.
- The tibial component is metal or polyethylene based and has a stem for fixation to bone.

Single-radius vs multi-radius

The total knee replacement implants are designed to match the geometry of bones as much as possible. In the past, the femoral component had a variable radius of curvature, on the basis that the posterior femoral condyles are elliptical when viewed from the side. However, the modern total knee replacements have a femoral component with a single radius of curvature in the sagittal plane, as the posterior femoral condyles are found to be circular when viewed from the side along the slanted flexion–extension (transepicondylar) axis of the knee. The single-radius total knee replacement design has a similar axis of rotation to that of the natural knee joint, which optimises the function of the collateral ligaments and other soft tissues of the knee. Therefore, it is considered to better replicate the normal motions of the natural knee joint.

Stability vs mobility

Total knee replacement prostheses can be classified according to their degree of 'constraint' to natural knee motion. This, in turn, is related to the design of the implants and depends on a number of factors, such as conformity of the bearing surfaces and features that substitute the function of supporting ligaments.

The range of motion of a natural or replacement joint is interconnected to its stability. In general, the more mobile a joint is, the less relatively stable it is and the more it relies on the surrounding soft tissues for stability. For example, the shoulder is the most mobile joint in the body, but is also most prone to dislocations and relies on its labrum and other soft tissues for stability; in comparison, although the hip is also a ball and socket joint, its motion is more constrained and the natural hip joint is far less prone to dislocations.

As a rule in total knee replacement, as the bearing surfaces become more conforming (i.e. matching) the prostheses gain more stability with less reliance on soft tissues. However, this is at the cost of increased constraint to motion. The selection of the type of implant design is therefore a compromise between its stability and mobility.

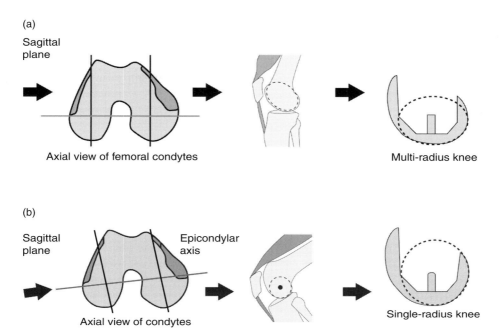

Fig. 7.9 Single-radius and multi-radius designs of femoral component. Medial and lateral collateral ligaments of the knee are inserted on the femur along the transepicondylar axis. The single-radius femoral component maintains natural tension in these ligaments throughout the flexion–extension arc. Clinical studies indicate that single-radius knee replacement provides better range of motion and improved overall functional results than multi-radius knee replacement. (Note: The transepicondylar axis is slanted in the axial plane, but is straight in the coronal plane as shown on page 113. It appears straight on page 125, because the whole femur is rotated.)

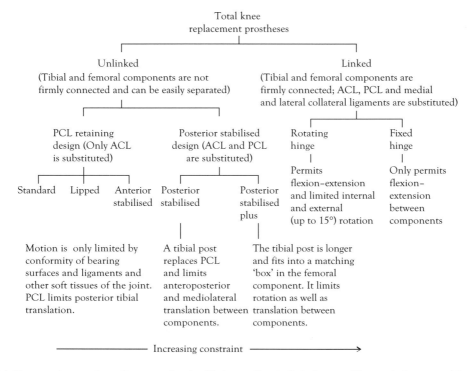

Fig. 7.10 Total knee replacement prostheses can be classified according to their degree of 'constraint' to natural knee motion. (ACL = anterior cruciate ligament; PCL = posterior cruciate ligament.)

Total knee replacement: design of components II

Fixed bearing vs mobile bearing

Total knee replacements have excellent long-term results, but a major limitation in their long-term survival is the wear of the polyethylene tibial insert. All designs of total knee replacement utilise metal (femoral component) on polyethylene (tibial insert) bearing combination. The tibial insert is the softer of the bearing surfaces and with time starts to wear, producing wear particles that lead to osteolysis and aseptic loosening at the bone–implant interface. Polyethylene wear is directly related to contact stresses generated on the tibial insert during relative motion between the bearing surfaces. Therefore, wear can be minimised by reducing contact stresses.

In the 'fixed bearing' total knee replacement design, the tibial insert is fixed to the tibial base plate. This prevents wear of the inferior surface of the tibial insert. The wear of the superior surface of the tibial insert is minimised by increasing its conformity to the femoral component, which increases the contact surface area and reduces contact stresses. An increase in conformity, however, also increases constraint to motion. This, in turn, leads to increased stresses at the bone–implant interface, which contributes to aseptic loosening.

The 'mobile bearing' knee replacement design offers an alternative solution to address the competing issues of wear, conformity and constraint. In this design, the tibial insert is mobile and not fixed to the tibial base plate. The wear of the superior surface of the tibial insert is minimised by the highly conforming interface with the femoral component, which distributes load over maximum contact area and therefore minimises contact stresses. The high conformity means that the motion at the interface is limited to flexion and extension only. However, axial rotation occurs at the interface between the inferior surface of the tibial insert and tibial base plate. Therefore, this design achieves high conformity without restricting axial rotation. A better range of motion at the bearing surfaces also reduces stresses at the bone–implant interface.

There are a number of limitations to the mobile bearing knee replacement design. Although the wear of the top surface of the tibial insert is minimised, there is added wear of the under-surface of the tibial insert, known as 'backside' wear. The wear particles are finer, and can more easily accumulate between the bone–implant interface. Therefore, the mobile bearing knee replacement design may even be at an increased risk of osteolysis and aseptic loosening. In addition, an increased motion between the interfaces makes it more prone to instability and dislocations. It is also not clear yet if the design produces a better range of motion clinically.

Patellar component

The patellar resurfacing component is circular and has a non-anatomical dome-shaped bearing surface. However, the convex shape is more tolerant of small degrees of patella mal-alignment. This design also eliminates the need to orientate the component.

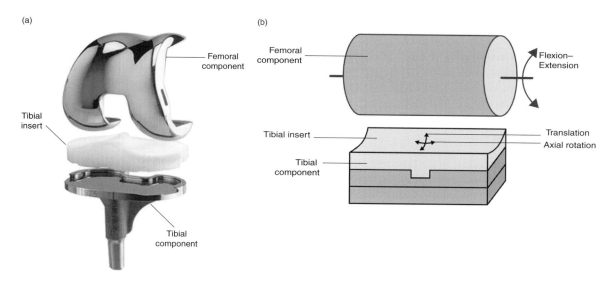

Fig. 7.11 In fixed bearing total knee replacement design, the tibial insert is fixed to the tibial component. All of the motion occurs at the interface between the femoral component and tibial insert. The superior surface of the tibial insert conforms to the shape of the femoral component. Although this increases the bearing surfaces' contact area, it also restricts axial rotation between them. (Image (a) is reproduced with permission of FH Orthopaedics.)

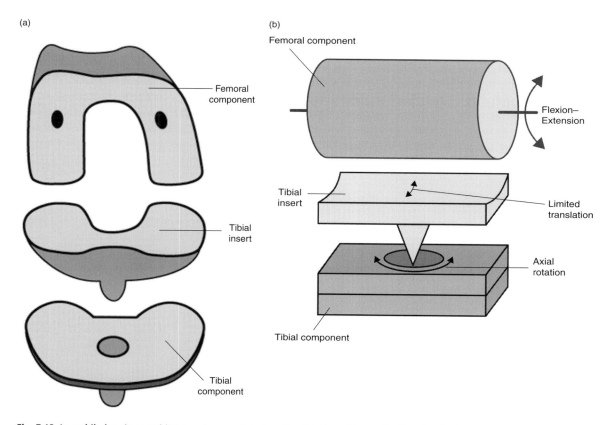

Fig. 7.12 In mobile bearing total knee replacement design, the tibial insert is not fixed to the tibial component. Flexion–extension occurs at the interface between the femoral component and tibial insert. The superior surface of the tibial insert is highly conforming to the shape of the femoral component. This ensures that the load is distributed over a maximum area. Axial rotation takes place at the interface between the tibial insert and the base plate.

Total knee replacement: alignment of components

The main biomechanical goals of knee replacement are to: maintain the mechanical axis of the lower limb; restore joint line and load-carrying capacity of the joint; and provide a functional range of movement with a well-fixed and durable prosthesis. The correct size and alignment of components and soft tissue balance are essential for a successful total knee replacement.

Femoral component

During flexion and extension of the knee, two aspects of the femoral condyles articulate with tibia: the distal condylar surface in knee extension and the posterior condylar surface in knee flexion. Both surfaces of the femur require correctly orientated cuts to achieve correct alignment of the femoral component in knee flexion and extension.

The distal femoral cut is made perpendicular to the mechanical axis. This ensures that the component is neutral with the mechanical axis and aligned with the centre of the femoral head. This is actually achieved by basing the cut on the femoral anatomical axis. As the mechanical axis is 5°–7° valgus to anatomical axis, a distal femoral cut 5°–7° valgus to the femoral anatomical axis is perpendicular to the mechanical axis.

The mechanical axis cannot be used to guide the posterior femoral cut, as the knee is in flexion. The posterior femoral cut is made parallel to the surgical epicondylar axis, which is defined as the line connecting the lateral epicondylar prominence with the medial epicondylar sulcus. A cut in this alignment results in 3° external rotation of the femoral component, which corresponds to the posterior slope of the tibial surface. The external rotation of the femoral component therefore ensures an equal gap between the bones in knee flexion. It is also important in restoring the correct Q-angle.

Tibial component

The proximal tibial cut is made perpendicular to mechanical axis of the tibia (which in practical terms is the same as its anatomical axis) to match with the distal femoral cut and ensure an equal gap between the bones in knee extension. The tibia is cut with about 3° posterior slope, unless the design of the implants accounts for the posterior slope.

The rotational alignment of the tibial component determines patella tracking. The internal rotation of the tibial component leads to external rotation of the tibial tubercle, which increases the Q-angle and the associated risk of patella subluxation and patella–femoral joint pain. The most reliable method for correct orientation of the tibial component is to align it with the medial third/border of the tibial tubercle.

Patellar component

Most of the complications after total knee replacement are related to the patellofemoral joint. The correct alignment of the femoral and tibial components is essential for normal patella tracking. The patellar implant is placed in a slightly medialised position, which ensures that the apex of the patella is in normal alignment. In some cases, the femoral implant can also be placed in a slightly lateral position, which relatively medialises the patella and improves patella tracking (Table 7.2).

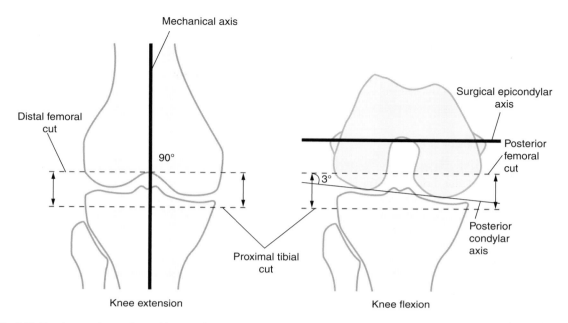

Fig. 7.13 The three main cuts in total knee replacement that determine the alignment of femoral and tibial components are distal and posterior femoral cuts and a proximal tibial cut. The other cuts involved in total knee replacement are: anterior femoral cut and anterior and posterior chamfer cuts – these shape the femur to match the geometry of the femoral component; and patellar cut to resurface the patella. Therefore, total knee replacement involves seven bone cuts.

Table 7.2. **Typical functional range of motion (degrees) required for some common everyday activities**

Activity	Hip joint	Knee joint
Level walking	−5–40	0–67
Ascending stairs	0–67	0–83
Descending stairs	0–35	0–90
Sitting down	0–105	0–110
Tying a shoelace*	0–125	0–106
Squatting**	0–117	0–130

* This has to be modified after total knee (and hip) replacement.

** Deep squatting is not possible/advisable after total knee (and hip) replacement.

Shoulder: functional anatomy I

The shoulder links the upper limb to the trunk. It is a complex of four joints: glenohumeral, acromioclavicular, sternoclavicular and scapulothoracic joints. The glenohumeral joint is the main joint of the shoulder complex, and is usually referred to as the shoulder joint. This chapter considers the biomechanics of the glenohumeral joint.

The glenohumeral joint is a ball and socket joint formed by the articulation of the head of the humerus with the glenoid of scapula.

Geometry and alignment of bones

The humeral head is retroverted 20°–30° with respect to the intercondylar plane of the distal humerus. This provides some restraint to anterior dislocation. The head–shaft angle is 130°–150°. Adjacent to the humeral head are the greater and lesser tuberosities, which are the attachment sites for ligaments and rotator cuff muscles.

The scapula is angled 30° anterior to the coronal plane – this is the 'plane of the scapula'. The scapula is also superiorly inclined 3°. The glenoid is retroverted 5° from the plane of the scapula and is superiorly inclined 5°. The superior inclination of the glenoid provides some restraint to inferior displacement of the humeral head.

The humeral head is approximately four times the size of the glenoid; this relationship is similar to that of a golf ball on a tee. As the humeral head is not that well 'covered' (constraint) by the glenoid, it can have a wide range of motion before structures on the opposite sides of the joint come into contact. As a result, the shoulder joint is the most mobile joint in the body. However, this lack of bony constraints also means that the joint is mainly dependent on other factors for stability. The key factors for shoulder stability are discussed below and in the next section.

Glenoid labrum

The glenoid is augmented by a rim of fibrocartilage, the glenoid labrum, which effectively doubles the depth of glenohumeral joint. The glenoid without the labrum encompasses about a quarter of the humeral head, but with the labrum this increases to a third of the humeral head. Although the overall joint contact area is relatively small, the articulating surfaces are highly congruent. The motion of the glenohumeral joint is therefore almost purely rotational. There is normally limited translation between the articulating surfaces. However, if the labrum is missing, abnormally formed or traumatically detached from the glenoid, there is loss of congruency between the articulating surfaces. This increases relative translation between the surfaces and therefore the risk of shoulder dislocation.

The three common structural abnormalities of the glenoid and labrum that can increase the risk of shoulder instability are as follows:

Bankart lesion: This is a traumatic detachment of anterior labrum from the glenoid.

Bony bankart lesion: This describes loss of a portion of glenoid with the anterior labrum.

SLAP tear: This is a superior labral tear from anterior to posterior (SLAP).

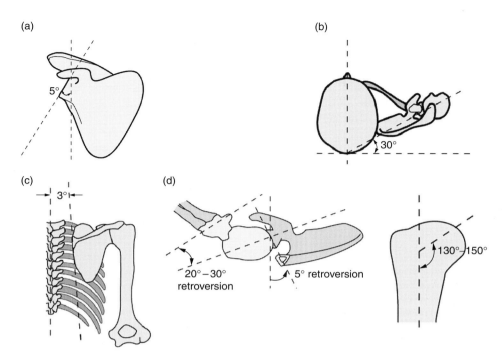

Fig. 8.1 **Geometry and alignment of bones forming the glenohumeral joint.**

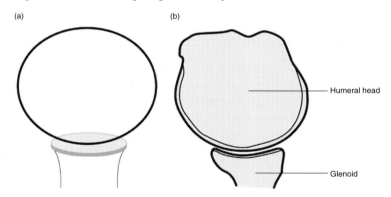

Fig. 8.2 **The glenohumeral joint is like a golf ball on a tee.** It is therefore a 'shallow' ball and socket joint. The humeral head is naturally inclined to 'fall off' i.e. dislocate. Most of the shoulder dislocations (90%–97%) are anterior.

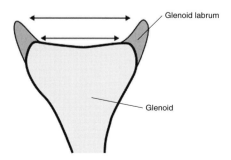

Fig. 8.3 **The glenoid labrum is an important stabiliser of the glenohumeral joint.** It increases the congruency between the articular surfaces. Bankart lesion, bony bankart lesion and SLAP tears are defects of the glenoid–labrum interface and can increase the risk of shoulder instability.

127

Shoulder: functional anatomy II

Joint capsule

The glenohumeral joint capsule is inherently lax and has twice the surface area of the humeral head. It is therefore quite flexible and permits a wide range of motion. However, different sections of the capsule tighten in different joint positions. Therefore, the capsule also contributes to joint stability. In frozen shoulder (adhesive capsulitis), there is contracture of the anterior aspect of the capsule, which reduces the overall motion of the joint, especially external rotation.

The capsule provides joint stability through a second mechanism. It maintains a negative intra-articular pressure, which pulls the capsule and the surrounding ligaments inwards. The closely adhered soft tissues prevent excessive translation between the articular surfaces and therefore reduce the risk of joint dislocation. A defect in the capsule or significant joint effusion greatly increases translation between articular surfaces.

Ligaments

There are three glenohumeral ligaments, which resist translation of the humeral head in different directions.
- The superior glenohumeral ligament is the primary restraint to inferior translation.
- The middle glenohumeral ligament is a restraint to anterior translation, being most effective in mid-abduction.
- The inferior glenohumeral ligament is the most dominant in maintaining joint stability. It consists of three portions: anterior band, axillary pouch and posterior band. The anterior band provides restraint to anterior translation when the arm is abducted and externally rotated. The posterior band provides restraint to posterior translation when the arm is abducted and internally rotated.

In addition, the coracohumeral ligament also resists inferior translation and external rotation of the humeral head.

Rotator cuff muscles

Rotator cuff muscles provide joint motion and stability. There are four rotator cuff muscles:
- supraspinatus assists deltoid in shoulder abduction
- subscapularis internally rotates the shoulder
- infraspinatus and teres minor externally rotate the shoulder.

The supraspinatus works with deltoid to produce a force couple (see pages 6–7) to abduct and forward flex the shoulder. The force of deltoid is directed mainly upwards and the force of supraspinatus is directed mainly medially. The resulting force couple rotates the humeral head and draws it medially into the glenoid.

Rotator cuff muscles provide stability by passive muscle tension and dynamic contraction. The importance of dynamic stability provided by the rotator cuff muscles is highlighted by the following example: it is difficult to abduct the arm fully with the palm facing towards the back but much easier with the palm facing forward. In the first case, supraspinatus and deltoid abduct the arm, but the impaction of greater tuberosity against acromium of the scapula halts the motion. In the second case, infraspinatus and teres minor rotate the humeral head externally, and together with supraspinatus and subscapularis draw the humeral head medially and inferiorly, allowing it to clear the acromium and achieve high abduction. The full arc of motion also requires rotation of the scapulothoracic joint.

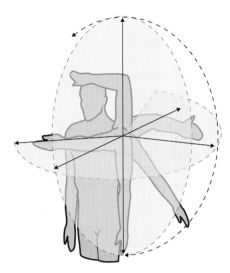

Fig. 8.4 The shoulder is the most mobile joint in the body. It allows up to 180° of forward flexion, 60° of extension (posterior elevation), 180° of abduction and 90° of internal and external rotation. The range of motion of shoulder normally decreases as part of the ageing process, although physical activity can counteract this process.

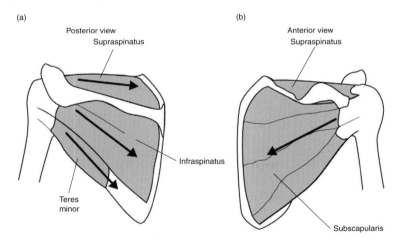

Fig. 8.5 There are four rotator cuff muscles: supraspinatus, infraspinatus, teres minor and subscapularis. The supraspinatus pulls mainly in a horizontal direction. The infraspinatus pulls approximately 45° and the teres minor pulls approximately 55° to the horizontal. Similarly, the subscapularis pulls approximately 45° to the horizontal.

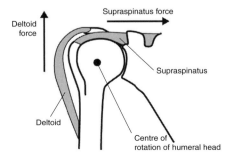

Fig. 8.6 The deltoid and supraspinatus produce a force couple to abduct and forward flex the shoulder. However, high shoulder abduction also requires obligatory external rotation of the humeral head. The rotator cuff muscles work together to draw the humeral head medially and inferiorly, allowing it to clear the acromium.

Shoulder joint reaction force

The shoulder joint reaction force depends on the position of the glenohumeral joint and the elbow joint. It is usually greatest when the shoulder is abducted to 90°. The calculations of exact joint reaction force are complex due to the large number of muscles active in any particular joint position. The following simplified static analyses highlight the effect of elbow extension and flexion on shoulder joint reaction force.

Shoulder abduction with elbow in extension

When the shoulder is in 90° of abduction, the deltoid contracts to maintain the position of the arm. The shoulder acts as the axis of a class III lever system; the muscles have a shorter lever arm than the weight of the arm. According to the static analysis, the minimum joint reaction force in this position is about one-half of total body weight.

Assumptions

In addition to the general assumptions, the following specific assumptions are applied to this static analysis:
- The deltoid provides all of the abduction force to stabilise the arm.
- The deltoid force is directed medially in a horizontal plane.
- The following physical measurements are based on anthropometric data:
  - The mass of the arm is approximately 5% total body mass. Therefore, in a 70 kg adult, the mass of the arm is assumed to be 3.5 kg. This equates to a weight of 35 N. This is assumed to act as a point load at the centre of weight of the arm, taken to be at the elbow joint, at 300 mm from the centre of rotation of the glenohumeral joint.
  - At 90° shoulder abduction, the moment arm of deltoid is 30 mm from the centre of rotation of the glenohumeral joint.

Shoulder abduction with elbow in flexion

Flexing the elbow moves the centre of weight of the arm closer to the body. Therefore, the abductor muscles have to produce less force to hold the arm in the abducted position. The static analysis shows that the joint reaction force now is about a quarter of total body weight.

Assumptions

As above, except:
- when the elbow is flexed, the centre of the weight of the arm is 150 mm from the centre of rotation of the glenohumeral joint.

Clinical implications

The deltoid muscle force and therefore shoulder joint reaction force are considerably less when the elbow is flexed than when it is extended. Therefore, shoulder rehabilitation exercises can be adapted according to the patient's functional level by changing the degree of elbow extension.

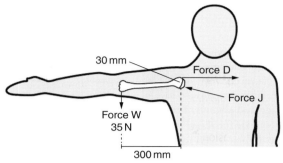

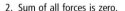

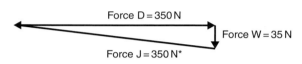

Fig. 8.7 Free-body force diagram of the upper limb showing the forces acting about the shoulder joint. The shoulder is abducted to 90° and the elbow is extended. (Force D = Deltoid force; Force W = Weight of the arm; and, Force J = Joint reaction force.)

Calculations

1. Sum of all moments is zero.

∴ Taking moments about the shoulder joint:
Total clockwise moments = Total anticlockwise moments
Force $D \times 0.03 = 35 \times 0.3$
Force $D = 350$ N

2. Sum of all forces is zero.

∴ A graphical method can be used to determine Force J.
Scale: 10 mm = 35 N.

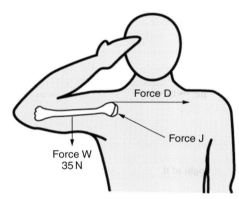

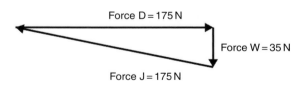

Fig. 8.8 Shoulder joint reaction force in abduction with elbow in extension. The joint reaction force is one-half of total body weight. **Free-body force diagram of the upper limb showing the forces acting about the shoulder joint.** The shoulder is abducted to 90° and the elbow is flexed.

Calculations

1. Sum of all moments is zero.

∴ Taking moments about the shoulder joint:
Total clockwise moments = Total anticlockwise moments
Force $D \times 0.03 = 35 \times 0.15$
Force $D = 175$ N

2. Sum of all forces is zero.

∴ A graphical method can be used to determine Force J.
Scale: 10 mm = 35 N.

Shoulder joint reaction force in abduction with elbow in flexion. The joint reaction force is a quarter of the total body weight.

*The arrow for Force J represents the magnitude and direction of the joint reaction force.

Shoulder replacement

Shoulder replacement is the third most common joint replacement. There are three forms of shoulder replacement:
- *Hemiarthroplasty* i.e. replacement of the humeral head only.
- *Total shoulder replacement*, i.e. replacement of the humeral head and glenoid.
- *Reversed shoulder replacement*, i.e. the bearing surfaces have an opposite profile to the normal anatomy.

This section takes a look at design and alignment of implants used in hemiarthroplasty and total shoulder replacement. The essential prerequisite for these 'conventional' procedures is that the rotator cuff is intact and functional. However, isolated small rotator cuff tears are compatible with these procedures. Non-functioning deltoid or rotator cuff are absolute contraindications to hemiarthroplasty and total shoulder replacement.

Humeral component

There are two main designs of humeral component: stemmed implant and resurfacing implant. The stemmed implant relies on intramedullary fixation and therefore has a cylindrical stem, which can be fixed to bone, either with or without cement. Cemented fixation immediately stabilises the component in the applied position. Therefore, cemented fixation is advantageous: when the bone quality is poor; when there is pre-existing bone deformity; or, when joint replacement is being performed for proximal humeral fractures, where the cement helps to stabilise fracture fragments as well as the implant. On the other hand, cementless fixation is also used widely as it avoids the problems associated with cemented fixation, especially the challenges of removing the implant and cement in revision surgery. Both types of stem are textured, and not smooth, for better interlocking with the surroundings. Cementless fixation stem in addition is porous coated in the proximal section to stimulate bone ingrowth for biological fixation. It is usually not coated along the whole length as this could make implant removal difficult in revision surgery. After the stem is satisfactorily fixed in the humerus, the appropriate size humeral head is applied to complete the component.

The resurfacing implant (shoulder resurfacing) only replaces the humeral joint surface and does not have an intramedullary stem. It therefore preserves bone stock and is easier to revise than the stemmed implant.

Glenoid component

This comprises an all-polyethylene implant, which has a concave articular surface and multiple pegs at the back for insertion into the bone. Most glenoid components are fixed with cement.

The glenoid is usually not affected by arthritis as much as the humeral head, and therefore does not always need to be replaced. It is usually only replaced when the chondral surface is completely worn out. The glenoid is usually well preserved and therefore not replaced in isolated osteonecrosis of the humeral head and proximal humeral fractures. Another reason for replacing glenoid selectively is that loosening of the glenoid component is one of the main causes of failure of the shoulder replacement. Therefore, there are inherent reservations about replacing the glenoid (Tables 8.1, 8.2).

(a)   (b)

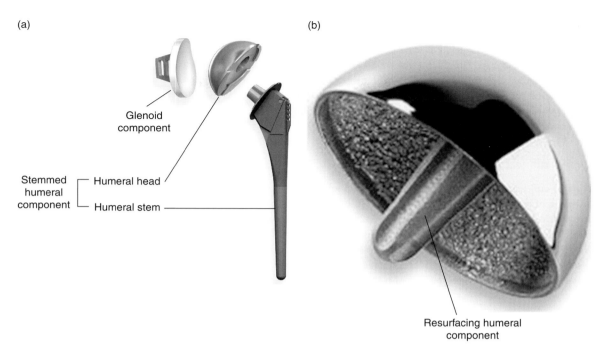

Glenoid
component

Stemmed   ┌─ Humeral head
humeral
component   └─ Humeral stem

Resurfacing humeral
component

Fig. 8.9 Types of implants used in shoulder replacement. The humeral component may be (a) stemmed or (b) resurfacing type. Both types of humeral component can be implanted without replacing the glenoid, as a hemiarthroplasty, or with the glenoid component, as a total shoulder replacement. Image (a) courtesy of Arthrex. Image (b) is reproduced with permission of Biomet. Biomet is the owner of the copyrights and all other intellectual property rights in relation to the image. Other than providing permission to use the image, this publication is not financially supported by Biomet.

Table 8.1. **Shoulder resurfacing**

Indications	Glenohumeral joint arthritis in younger, more active patients – they are more likely to require a revision procedure.
	Proximal humerus deformity.
	Rotator cuff tears.
	Previous fractures of the humerus that have been internally fixed with a nail or a plate – it may be possible not to disturb previously implanted metalwork by performing shoulder resurfacing.
Advantages	Does not involve humeral neck osteotomy, therefore head–shaft angle does not need to be addressed.
	Involves minimal bone resection.
	Shorter operation time.
	Lower risk of periprosthetic fractures.
	Easier revision to a conventional shoulder replacement.
Contra-indications	Severe osteoporosis – as the bone would not be able to support the component.
	Proximal humeral fracture – this would require a stemmed prosthesis.

Table 8.2. **Alignment of components**

The humeral head is implanted in 25–45° retroversion and with a head–shaft angle more than 130°. Varus placement must be avoided as the loads acting on the component are pushing the implant in this direction. The glenoid component is usually implanted in neutral alignment with respect to the plane of the scapula.

Reversed shoulder replacement

Reversed shoulder arthroplasty is used in patients with non-functional rotator cuff muscles. The two most common indications for reversed shoulder replacement are rotator cuff tear arthropathy and massive, irreparable rotator cuff tear (even without established arthritis). Other indications include: rheumatoid arthritis, which is usually associated with rotator cuff dysfunction; revision for failed hemiarthroplasty or total shoulder replacement associated with rotator cuff damage; and displaced comminuted proximal humerus fractures where anatomical alignment of standard components may be difficult.

Rotator cuff tear arthropathy

Rotator cuff tear arthropathy is the glenohumeral joint arthritis secondary to chronic massive rotator cuff tear. The function of rotator cuff muscles is to stabilise the humeral head, which includes preventing it from translating superiorly during abduction (see pages 128–129). However, a massive tear in the rotator cuff tendon leaves the muscles effectively non-functional. As a result, the superiorly directed deltoid force acts unopposed. In addition, the long head of biceps is usually also torn in massive rotator cuff tear, and its normal humeral head depressing effect is also lost. The humeral head therefore migrates superiorly and wears against the superior aspect of the glenoid and the under-surface of the acromium. This also leads to erosion of the superior aspect of the glenoid.

Design of components

The humeral component is a stemmed implant with a polyethylene cup. The stem can be fixed to bone with the cemented or cementless method. The humeral component has a non-anatomical head–shaft angle of 155°.

The glenoid component consists of a large metal hemispherical ball (glenosphere) attached to a metal base plate. The base plate is fixed to the glenoid with screws, i.e. the cementless method. The humeral cup covers less than half of the glenosphere.

Mechanics of reversed shoulder replacement

The reversed relationship of the bearing surfaces has two important mechanical effects:
- It translates the centre of rotation medially and distally. A medial centre of rotation lengthens the lever arm of deltoid, so it works more effectively in the absence of assistance from supraspinatus. It also allows more deltoid fibres to be recruited for abduction and elevation. Therefore, a larger fraction of deltoid works more effectively to produce shoulder motion. The centre of rotation is, in fact, at the glenoid bone–prosthesis fixation interface. This reduces the torque on glenoid component. Therefore, the risk of glenoid component loosening in reversed shoulder replacement is less compared with conventional total shoulder replacement.
- It lowers the humerus relative to the glenoid. This increases tension in deltoid and further improves its performance.

As a result, reversed shoulder replacement reduces shear force and increases compressive forces across the joint.

The main limitation of reversed shoulder arthroplasty is that it is generally unable to restore the lost external rotation, which is caused by infraspinatus and teres minor deficiency.

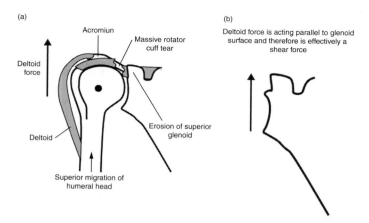

Fig. 8.10 Rotator cuff tear arthropathy is the glenohumeral joint arthritis secondary to chronic massive rotator cuff tear. In the absence of normally functioning rotator cuff muscles, the deltoid force acts as a shear force with respect to the glenoid, and draws the humeral head superiorly. This leads to wear of the humeral head and superior glenoid.

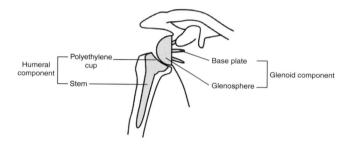

Fig. 8.11 Reversed shoulder replacement utilises a convex glenoid component and concave humeral component. Conventional shoulder replacement prostheses are unconstrained and rely on rotator cuff muscles for stability. However, reversed shoulder replacement prosthesis is semi-constrained and is further stabilised by non-anatomical head–shaft angle of the humeral component, and therefore does not rely on rotator cuff for stability.

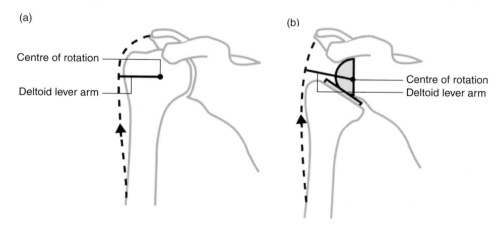

Fig. 8.12 Reversed shoulder arthroplasty translates the centre of rotation medially and distally, so that it lies at the glenoid bone–prosthesis interface. This provides the following mechanical advantages: lengthening of deltoid lever arm; recruitment of more deltoid fibres for elevation and abduction; and reduced torque on the glenoid component. It also lowers the humerus compared with the glenoid, which tensions the deltoid.

Elbow: functional anatomy

The elbow increases the flexibility of the upper limb. It also transmits forces between the arm and the forearm and acts as the axis for the forearm lever system. The elbow is a complex of three joints of humerus, ulna and radius: humeroulnar, humeroradial and proximal radioulnar joints. All three joints are enclosed within the same capsule.

The distal humerus is divided into medial and lateral columns, which are tilted anteriorly approximately 40° from the humeral shaft. The columns form two articulating surfaces at the elbow joint: capitellum and trochlea.

The humeroulnar joint is a hinge joint formed by the hourglass-shaped trochlea articulating with the saddle-shaped trochlea notch of the ulna. This is an inherently stable configuration, and restricts undue relative motion between the articulating surfaces. The humeroradial joint is a ball and socket joint. It is an unconstrained joint formed between capitellum, which is an almost perfect hemisphere, and radial head, which has little contact with the capitellum. The proximal radioulnar joint is a pivot joint formed by articulation between the adjacent surfaces of the radius and ulna. It is a relatively constrained joint.

Range of motion

The elbow joint complex allows two types of motion: flexion and extension occur at the humeroulnar and humeroradial joints; and pronation and supination occur at the humeroradial and proximal radioulnar joints, and also require simultaneous motion at the distal radioulnar joint. The two types of motion are independent of each other. The normal range of flexion–extension is 0°–140°, and pronation–supination is 75° pronation – 85° supination. The functional range of flexion–extension is 30°–120°, and pronation–supination is 50° pronation – 50° supination.

The primary flexors of the elbow are brachialis and biceps brachii. The brachialis is the main flexor of the elbow, and is also described as the 'workhorse' in elbow flexion. The biceps brachii is most effective as a flexor when the forearm is in supination; its main function is supination of the forearm. The brachialis and biceps brachii together produce more than 60% of elbow flexion force. The main extensor of the elbow is triceps brachii. Elbow pronation is produced by pronator teres and pronator quadratus and supination by biceps brachii and supinator.

Cubitus angle

When the elbow is in full extension and supination, the longitudinal axis of the forearm is valgus to the longitudinal axis of the arm. The angle formed between these two axes is called the cubitus or carrying angle. The carrying angle allows the forearm to clear the hip when the upper limb is swinging, such as during walking. The normal range for the carrying angle is between 10° and 15°. It is less in children than adults, and gradually increases with age. The carrying angle is generally greater in females than males, because females on average have smaller shoulders and wider hips. The carrying angle decreases with elbow flexion.

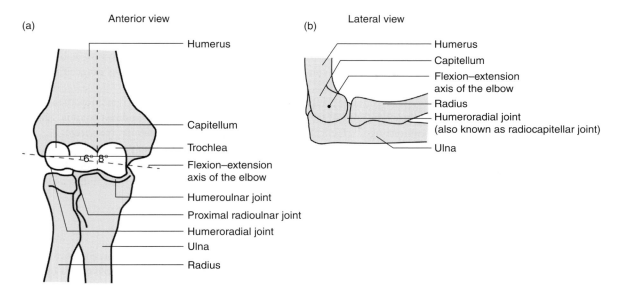

(a) Anterior view

Humerus

Capitellum

Trochlea

Flexion–extension axis of the elbow

Humeroulnar joint

Proximal radioulnar joint

Humeroradial joint

Ulna

Radius

(b) Lateral view

Humerus

Capitellum

Flexion–extension axis of the elbow

Radius

Humeroradial joint (also known as radiocapitellar joint)

Ulna

Fig. 9.1 The elbow is a complex of three joints of humerus, ulna and radius. The flexion–extension axis lies in the trochlea. In the coronal plane, it is 4°–8° valgus to the plane perpendicular to the longitudinal axis of the humerus. In the sagittal plane, it lies at the centre of the trochlea. The flexion–extension axis varies slightly at the extremes of motion. The elbow joint therefore is not a simple hinge but instead is described as a modified hinge.

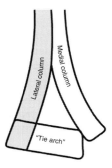

Lateral column

Medial column

"Tie arch"

Fig. 9.2 Mechanically, the distal humerus has the configuration of two columns joined together by a tie arch (trochlea).

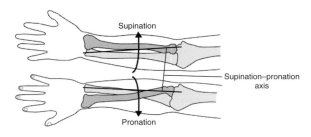

Supination

Supination–pronation axis

Pronation

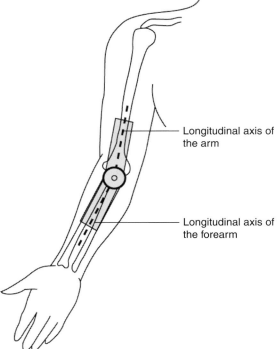

Longitudinal axis of the arm

Longitudinal axis of the forearm

Fig. 9.4 Supination–pronation axis passes through the centre of the capitellum of the distal humerus, the radial head and the distal ulna head. Therefore, it is not parallel to the longitudinal axis of the forearm.

Fig. 9.3 The carrying angle is clinically measured as the angle between the longitudinal axis of the arm and forearm. It results from the fact that the trochlea extends distal to the capitellum, and therefore the longitudinal axis of the ulna is, on average, 6° valgus to the longitudinal axis of the humerus.

Stabilisers of the elbow

The elbow joint complex derives its stability equally from bony and soft tissues components. The arrangement of three joints together producing the two main arcs of motion is a unique way of balancing motion with stability; although each joint is relatively constrained, the joint complex as a whole still produces a generous range of motion. As a result, the elbow joint complex is overall inherently stable.

The elbow, however, is the second most dislocated joint in the body (after the shoulder). This is an indication of the magnitude of forces transmitted to the elbow joint in falls onto the outstretched hand and in direct trauma. Elbow dislocation is associated with two contrasting mechanical complications: stiffness and instability (recurrent dislocations). Elbow stiffness usually develops after a prolonged period of immobilisation to prevent instability. Therefore, a proper assessment of elbow stability is important at the outset in order to plan the correct treatment.

The structures that provide elbow stability can be classified as static or dynamic stabilisers.

Static stabilisers

Static stabilisers are further divided into primary or secondary stabilisers.

The primary static stabilisers are the humeroulnar joint and medial and lateral collateral ligament complexes. The humeroulnar joint is a constraint joint due to the congruency of the articulating surfaces. The stable nature of the large humeroulnar joint stabilises the whole elbow unit.

The ligaments provide further stability to the elbow joint complex. The medial collateral ligament complex consists of three bands: anterior, posterior and transverse. The anterior band is the primary restraint to valgus stress. If the anterior band is disrupted, the radial head, i.e. humeroradial joint, acts as a secondary stabiliser against valgus stress. A radial head fracture in the presence of an intact anterior band usually does not cause instability.

The humeroulnar articulation (especially coronoid process) provides the main resistance to varus stress. The lateral collateral ligament complex is the main soft tissue restraint to varus stress; however, it has a minor role towards varus stability. The main function of the lateral collateral ligament complex is restraint to posterolateral rotatory instability. It consists of four individual ligaments: radial collateral ligament, lateral ulnar collateral ligament, annular ligament and accessory collateral ligament. The lateral ulna collateral ligament and radial collateral ligament are the primary restraints to posterolateral rotatory instability.

The joint capsule acts as a secondary stabiliser to limit excessive motion in all directions. The tendons of the common flexors and extensors in the forearm are also secondary stabilisers. The interosseous membrane between the ulna and radius is also a stabiliser of the elbow joint complex, as it maintains the relative position of the two bones and prevents longitudinal instability.

Dynamic stabilisers

The muscles that cross the joint, e.g. triceps, biceps and brachialis, generate stabilising compressive forces that provide dynamic stability to the elbow joint complex (Table 9.1).

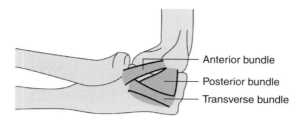

Fig. 9.5 Anatomy of the medial collateral ligament complex. The anterior band is the main restraint to valgus instability; it is the stiffest and strongest of all the ligaments of the elbow joint. The anterior band is tightened in flexion and the posterior band is tightened in extension. The transverse bundle does not span a joint and therefore does not contribute to elbow stability.

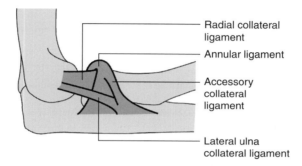

Fig. 9.6 Anatomy of the lateral collateral ligament complex. The lateral ulna collateral ligament and radial collateral ligament are the primary restraints to posterolateral rotatory instability. The annular ligament encompasses the radial head and holds the proximal radioulna joint together.

Table 9.1. **Elbow stability: clinical perspective**

A primary stabiliser is a structure which, if deficient, leads to instability. A secondary stabiliser is a structure which, if deficient, on its own does not cause instability. However, a deficiency of a secondary stabiliser when the primary stabiliser is also compromised worsens the resultant instability.

Elbow dislocations are classified as simple, when there is no associated fracture, or complex, when there are associated fractures around the elbow. A simple elbow dislocation causes injury to the ligaments (and joint capsule), usually in a circular pattern from lateral to medial. Despite the ligamentous injury, elbow stability is usually maintained by the dynamic structures. Therefore, most patients with simple elbow dislocation are treated functionally with protected early active motion exercises whilst the injured ligaments heal. However, a ligamentous injury that results in gross instability during functional arc of motion or chronic instability (recurrent dislocations) usually requires surgical repair of the injured ligaments. The management of a complex elbow dislocation depends on the associated fracture and the resultant instability. The term 'terrible triad' describes the combination of elbow dislocation and fracture of the radial head and coronoid process. This is associated with a high risk of complications.

Elbow joint reaction force

Flexion

When the elbow is held at 90° of flexion by the side of the body, the brachialis is the main muscle that maintains this position of the forearm. According to the static analysis, the elbow joint reaction force in this position is more than one and a half times the weight of the supported forearm (see pages 10–11 for full analysis).

Extension

In this case, the elbow is held at 90° of flexion with the forearm positioned above the head. Now, the triceps brachii is contracting to maintain the position of the forearm. The static analysis shows that the elbow joint reaction force is more than five times the weight of the supported forearm.

Assumptions

In addition to the general assumptions, the following specific assumptions are applied to this static analysis.

- The triceps brachii provides all of the extension force.
- The triceps brachii generates a downward force only.
- The following physical measurements are based on anthropometric data.
  - Forearm weight is 15 N, and is assumed to act as a point load at the centre of weight of the forearm, 130 mm from the centre of rotation of the joint (see pages 10–11 for details).
  - At 90° elbow flexion, the insertion point of triceps brachii is 30 mm from the centre of rotation of the joint.

Discussion

The elbow joint reaction force during extension is more than three times during flexion. This is because the lever arm of the triceps brachii (30 mm) is shorter than that of brachialis (50 mm). Therefore, muscular and joint reaction forces produced during elbow extension are much greater than during flexion.

The moment arms of the muscles acting at the elbow joint change with elbow flexion angle. The moment arm of the brachialis increases with elbow flexion. It is the longest at approximately 100° of flexion, and shortens slightly with further flexion. At the same time, the moment arm of the weight of the forearm also increases with elbow flexion, and starts to decrease after 90° of flexion. The brachialis is more effective during the second half of the flexion–extension arc than during the first half. Similarly, the moment arm of the triceps brachii is shortest when the elbow is in full flexion, and progressively increases with extension.

Although the elbow joint is considered to be a non-weight-bearing joint, it still experiences significant forces during everyday activities. The elbow joint force is estimated to be 300 N when eating and dressing, 1700 N when using the arms to rise from a chair and 1900 N when pulling a table across the floor. The joint force can reach up to three times total body weight during certain activities.

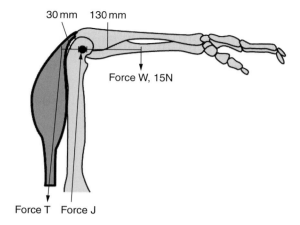

30 mm 130 mm

Force W, 15N

Force T   Force J

Fig. 9.7 Free-body force diagram of the upper limb showing forces acting about the elbow joint during extension. The elbow is held at 90° of flexion. It is acting as the axis of a class I lever. The moment arm of muscles is shorter than that of the weight of the forearm. (Force T = Triceps force; Force W = Weight of the forearm; and, Force J = Joint reaction force.)

Calculations

Applying the conditions of equilibrium:

1. Sum of all moments is zero.

∴ Taking moments about the elbow joint:
Total clockwise moments = Total anticlockwise moments
$$15 \times 0.13 = \text{Force } T \times 0.03$$
$$\text{Force } T = 65 \text{ N}$$

2. Sum of all forces is zero.

∴ Force J + (−Force T) + (−Force W) = 0
$$\text{Force } J - 65 - 15 = 0$$
$$\text{Force } J = 80 \text{ N}$$

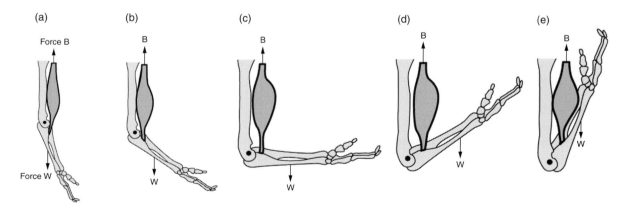

(a) (b) (c) (d) (e)

Force B

B   B   B   B

Force W

W   W   W   W

Elbow joint reaction force during extension. The joint reaction force is more than five times the weight of the forearm.

Fig. 9.8 The moment arms of brachialis and weight of the forearm vary with elbow flexion angle. Similarly, the moment arm of triceps also varies with elbow flexion angle. (Force B = Brachialis force; Force W = Weight of the forearm.)

Biomechanics of spinal components I

The spinal column is designed to carry loads and provide a wide range of movements, whilst also protecting the spinal cord and the related neurovascular structures.

The vertebrae provide stiffness to the spinal column.

Vertebrae

A typical vertebra has the following common key features: vertebral body, facet (intervertebral) joints, and spinous and transverse processes.

Vertebral body

The vertebral body is the main load-bearing part of the vertebra. It is designed to support mainly compressive loads, which are produced by the weight of the body above the vertebra. A typical vertebral body has the shape of a short cylinder. It has a thin shell of cortical bone surrounding a core of porous cancellous bone. The cancellous bone is organised into vertical and horizontal trabaculae, which is the most effective arrangement to resist compressive force. The compressive force is resisted mainly by the vertical 'columns', and the horizontal 'cross-beams' prevent the columns from bowing under stress. This arrangement of cancellous bone converts an axial compressive force into a transverse tensile force. The fact that vertebrae are not solidly filled with bone is also mechanically important. Solid vertebrae would be significantly heavier and less effective at withstanding dynamic loads. This is because solid structures are less 'springy' and provide less 'cushion' when loaded suddenly (hence the reason why empty cardboard boxes can be used to cushion a person falling from a height). The porous cancellous bone enables the vertebrae to be lightweight and still be adequately stiff and strong to withstand different types of loads.

The most common injury of the spinal column is compression fracture of the vertebral body. It usually occurs in osteoporosis, where supporting framework of cancellous bone is not as extensive as normal. It can also occur in high-energy injuries where the applied compressive force exceeds the strength of the normal vertebral body.

The vertebral bodies have smooth surfaces and therefore cannot control relative motion between each other. They are completely dependent on other structures for stability in the transverse plane.

Facet joints

The facet joints guide motion between adjacent vertebrae. The orientation of the facet joint changes between the spinal segments; therefore, different segments have different profiles of motion. The facet joints also have a load-bearing function. They share the load transmitted between the vertebrae with the intervertebral disc. The proportion of load shared by facet joints and intervertebral disc varies with the position of the spine. They normally carry up to 30% of the transmitted load.

Spinous and transverse processes

The spinous and transverse processes provide areas for attachment of ligaments and muscles. They provide lever arms to ligaments and muscles, and therefore reduce the force required from them to maintain function.

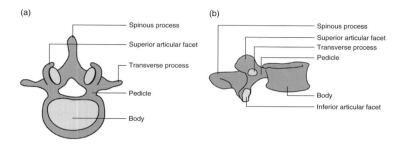

Fig. 10.1 The anatomy of a lumbar vertebra.

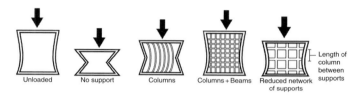

Fig. 10.2 Bucking strength of a structure is proportional to the number of columns supporting it and the length of column between supports. The vertebral body consists of a thin outer layer of cortical bone supported by an extensive scaffold of cancellous bone. Osteoporosis reduces the bone density and weakens the supporting framework.

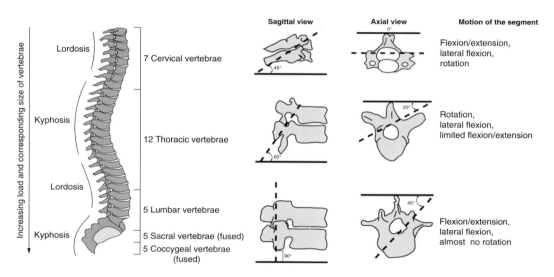

Fig. 10.3 Humans are the only mammals that have a vertebral column with four curves in the sagittal plane. These curves are a feature of bipedal locomotion, and increase the flexibility and load-bearing capacity of the spinal column. The orientation of facet joints of the vertebrae changes between the spinal segments; therefore, different segments have different profiles of motion.

Biomechanics of spinal components II

The discs and ligaments provide flexibility to the spinal column.

Intervertebral disc

An intervertebral disc consists of three structures: nucleus pulposus in the centre, annulus fibrosis on the outside and vertebral end plates at the top and bottom. The nucleus pulposus has a high water content and generates hydrostatic pressure. The annulus fibrosis consists of concentric layers of collagen fibres. Hydrostatic pressure in the nucleus pulposus creates tensile stress in annulus fibrosis, which provides stiffness to the disc.

The vertebral end plate is a cartilage structure that connects the disc to the adjacent vertebrae. It allows diffusion of nutrients and waste products between the disc and blood vessels in the vertebral bone marrow.

The intervertebral disc acts as a shock absorber and provides movement in the 'functional spinal unit'. When the disc is loaded, hydrostatic pressure increases in the nucleus pulposus. The nucleus pulposus exerts this pressure against the surrounding annulus fibrosus, in accordance with Pascal's law, which states that pressure within a fluid is transmitted equally in all directions. The annulus fibrosus expands in the transverse plane and shortens in the vertical plane. This change in shape of the intervertebral disc converts axial stress into circumferential stress, which is also known as tensile hoop stress. This process reduces the load transmitted between the vertebrae. Under prolonged loading, the intervertebral disc experiences further deformation due to outflow of fluid from the vertebral end plates. In mechanical terms, this is described as creep, i.e. time-dependent deformation under constant load. The intervertebral disc therefore is a viscoelastic material. Disc deformation is recovered when the applied load is removed. This leads to diurnal variation in a person's height: a person is usually slightly taller in the morning compared with the evening.

Disc degeneration leads to mechanical failure of the intervertebral disc. It starts with loss of hydration of nucleus pulposus. As the nucleus pulposus becomes less turgid, collagen layers of annulus fibrosis delaminate, collapse inwards and develop concentric tears. This is associated with loss of disc height, which leads to subluxation of the facet joints. The facet joints begin to transmit increased loads (up to 70% of total transmitted load) and as a result develop degenerative changes. Disc degeneration therefore affects load transfer and movements of the functional spinal unit.

Ligaments and muscles

The ligaments hold the vertebrae and intervertebral discs together. The stiffness of ligaments increases up to 75 times outside the normal range of motion. Therefore, the spinal column has high flexibility in the 'elastic zone' of ligaments, but has to overcome much higher resistance to exceed the safe limits of motion. The muscles act to stabilise and create movement in the spinal column.

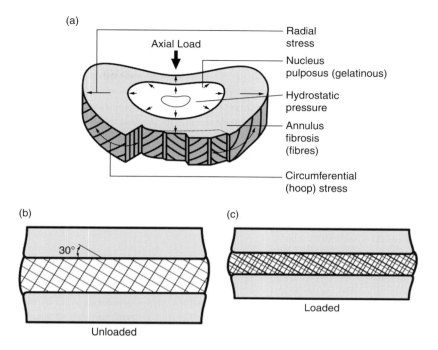

Fig. 10.4 An intervertebral disc acts as a shock absorber and provides movement in the functional spinal unit. It is the largest avascular structure in the body, and relies on vertebral end plates for metabolic support. (a) When it is loaded, the nucleus pulposus exerts uniform hydrostatic pressure on the surrounding annulus fibrosis. (b) The collagen fibres of the annulus fibrosis are arranged 30° to the vertebral end plate, alternating in direction between layers. This is the optimal arrangement for withstanding both the tensile forces generated by nucleus pulposus and the shear forces produced by relative motion between the vertebrae. (c) The fibres flatten out when the disc is loaded. The change in the shape of the disc produces circumferential 'hoop' stress. This process reduces the load transmitted to the underlying vertebrae.

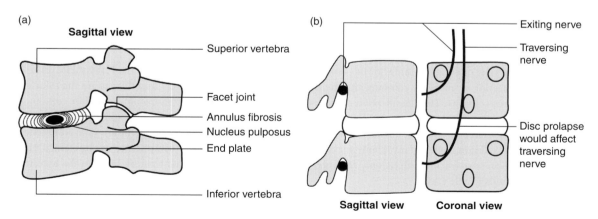

Fig. 10.5 The functional spinal unit is the shortest segment of spine that has the same biomechanical properties as the whole vertebral column. It is also described as the spinal motion segment. (a) It consists of two adjacent vertebrae, an intervertebral disc and the associated ligaments. Motion in the functional spinal unit occurs at three joints: the two facet joints and the intervertebral joint.
(b) The relationship of the intervertebral disc with exiting and traversing spinal nerves. A nerve exits above the disc, therefore a disc prolapse would normally affect the traversing nerve and not the exiting nerve. However, if a disc prolapsed into a 'far lateral' position, it would affect the exiting nerve.

Stability of the spinal column

The spinal column has a wide range of motion: flexion, extension, lateral flexion and axial rotation. This large overall flexibility is achieved by small displacements at each spinal motion segment. The vertebrae have six degrees of freedom motion: they can translate along and about in the axial, sagittal and coronal planes. Therefore, the overall motion of the spinal column is produced by a combination of translation and rotation of individual vertebrae. It is important that the displacement at each motion segment does not exceed the normal limits, as this could potentially result in a neurological injury, significant deformity or intolerable mechanical pain.

The spinal column is considered to be mechanically stable when normal loading does not cause excessive displacement of the spinal motion segment. In the setting of a spinal injury, one of the most important clinical tasks is to determine whether the spinal column is stable. Two conventional classification systems of spinal stability are based on the integrity of spinal column structures in the sagittal profile. Both classification systems are related to the thoraco-lumbar regions.

Two-column classification (Holdworth, 1960)

According to this classification, the spinal column is made of two individual columns:
- The anterior column consists of anterior longitudinal ligament, vertebral body, intervertebral disc and posterior longitudinal ligament.
- The posterior column consists of the pedicles, facet joints, transverse and spinous processes and the associated ligaments.

A traumatic disruption of both columns leads to spinal instability and a significant risk of injury to neurovascular structures. If only one column is disrupted, then spinal stability depends on the integrity of the ligaments supporting the affected column. Any associated subluxation (to any degree) indicates disruption of supporting ligaments and therefore instability. The classification proposes that spinal stability relies mainly on the posterior column structures.

Three-column classification (Denis, 1983)

This classification considers the spinal column in terms of three individual columns:
- The anterior column consists of the anterior longitudinal ligament and the anterior half of the vertebral body and intervertebral disc.
- The middle column consists of the posterior longitudinal ligament and the posterior half of the vertebral body and intervertebral disc.
- The posterior column, as in the two-column classification, consists of the pedicles, facet joints, transverse and spinous processes and the associated ligaments.

Isolated disruptions of either the anterior or posterior columns (i.e. one column) are mechanically stable. Injuries that affect the anterior or posterior columns *and* the middle column are mechanically unstable, as are the injuries that affect all three columns. The classification proposes that spinal stability relies mainly on the middle column. Biomechanical studies confirm that the middle column is indeed the primary determinant of spinal stability. However, this is not an anatomically distinct zone, and isolated injuries of the middle column are rare. In practical terms, the middle column is important mainly for distinguishing between a purely compressive fracture and a burst fracture: the compressive fracture affects only the anterior column whereas the burst fracture involves the anterior and middle columns (Table 10.1).

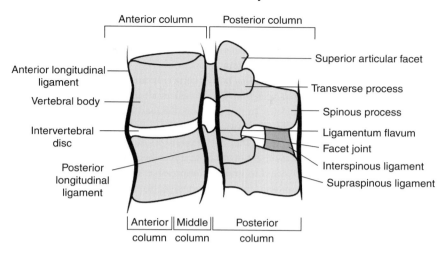

Two-column theory

Anterior column | Posterior column

Anterior longitudinal ligament
Vertebral body
Intervertebral disc
Posterior longitudinal ligament

Superior articular facet
Transverse process
Spinous process
Ligamentum flavum
Facet joint
Interspinous ligament
Supraspinous ligament

Anterior column | Middle column | Posterior column

Three-column theory

Fig. 10.6 The two-column and three-column classifications of spinal injuries. The stability of the spinal column relies on the interplay between bony and soft tissue structures. A column is disrupted when any of the structures in the column are affected.

Table 10.1. **Spinal stability: clinical perspective**

In the setting of an acute spinal injury, the Advanced Trauma Life Support (ATLS) protocol should be used to stabilise, examine, investigate and manage the patient. The stability of the spinal column is evaluated by clinical assessment and appropriate radiological investigations. It is essential to perform a full neurological examination. Focal signs around the spinal column (e.g. swelling, bruising and tenderness) may indicate underlying ligamentous or bony injury. Plain radiographs are useful to check for obvious structural abnormalities. Computer tomography (CT) scan provides further details on the extent of bony injuries and any compromise of the spinal canal. Magnetic resonance imaging (MRI) scan is useful to assess the soft tissues, such as the ligaments, intervertebral disc and spinal cord. Sometimes, dynamic radiographs may be required to evaluate spinal stability, e.g. standing radiographs after application of a brace for a vertebral fracture that initially appears stable.

The spinal column is considered to be mechanically stable when the initial injury is not likely to cause excessive displacement of the spinal motion segment when the patient bears weight. However, a mechanically stable spinal column may not be neurologically stable. It may be neurologically unstable due to initial injury from fracture fragments, a herniated intervertebral disc, epidural haematoma or a compromise in blood supply to the spinal cord.

The management of a patient with spinal instability depends on the underlying cause and whether there is associated neurological compromise. A patient with a mechanically and neurologically unstable spine may require surgical intervention, e.g. decompression of neurological structures with or without surgical stabilisation. On the other hand, a patient with vertebral fractures and no neurological compromise may be treated with bed rest until the fractures are healed. Generally, it is difficult to improve a neurologically stable patient or to reverse neurological deficit in a patient who has developed flaccid paralysis.

The loads acting on the spinal column

The cervical and lumbar segments of the spinal column are the most mobile. Therefore, degenerative changes are also most common in these segments. The loads acting on the spine increase at each lower level, making the lumbar segment subject to the greatest loads. This section considers the loads produced in the lumbar segment, to provide an appreciation of the peak loads found in the spinal column.

The loads acting on the spinal column are affected by body posture. In an upright standing position, the centre of body weight lies anterior to the fourth lumbar vertebra. This produces a forwards moment on the spinal column, which is balanced by spinal ligaments and muscles. In this position, the load acting on the intervertebral disc between the third and fourth vertebrae is estimated to be about twice the weight of the body above this level. The material and geometric properties of the intervertebral disc mean that the pressure within the disc is approximately 1½ times the applied stress. Forward flexion increases the moment arm of the upper body weight and the resultant loads on the functional spinal unit. The vertebrae are subjected to mainly compressive loads even in variable positions. However, the intervertebral discs are subjected to a combination of compressive, bending and torsional loads, which increase with movements of the spinal column.

In a classical experiment, invasive pressure monitoring was used in healthy volunteers (medical students) to measure pressures in the disc between the third and fourth vertebrae in various body positions. The study found that intradiscal pressures were greater when sitting than when standing. In both cases, the intradiscal pressures increased on forward flexion and carrying external loads. Another similar study found that intradiscal pressures in the sitting position were reduced with the use of a lumbar support ('supported sitting') and also in a reclined position.

The vertebral column, in evolutionary terms, is not designed for prolonged periods of sitting down. However, this is quite common in modern life, and is considered to contribute to lower back complaints. A person with acute back pain may find that symptoms exacerbate when sitting, and should lie flat to offload the intervertebral discs. The loads acting on the spinal column are minimised when lying flat because loads produced by the body weight are eliminated. However, tension in the psoas muscles – which originate from transverse processes of thoracic and lumbar vertebrae – causes some residual loading of the lumbar segment. This can be minimised by lifting the legs on a support so that the hips and knees are flexed, which relaxes the psoas muscles.

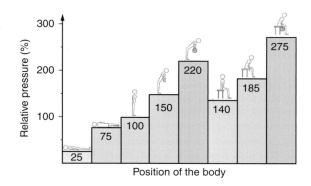

Fig. 10.7 Relative pressure in the disc between third and fourth vertebrae measured in different body positions. Intradiscal pressure in standing position is taken as 100%. (These findings were reported in the following textbook: White AP, Panjabi MM (eds) (1990). *Clinical Biomechanics of the Spine.* Philadelphia: Lippincott, Williams & Wilkins.)

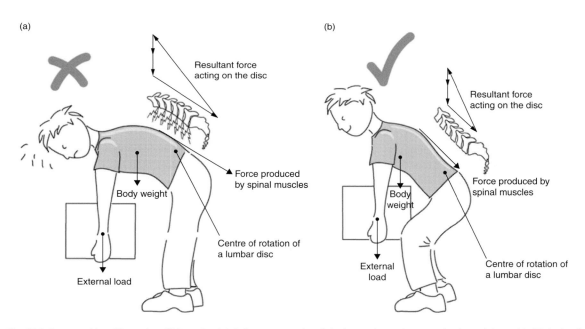

Fig. 10.8 In manual handling, when lifting a load, it is important to bend the knees, keep the upper back straight and hold the load close to the body. These measures reduce the forward moments produced by the body weight and external load, which reduces the force produced by spinal muscles and the resultant force acting on the lumbar intervertebral discs.

The ankle joint

Functional anatomy

The ankle is a unit of two joints: the talocrural joint, which is usually referred to as the ankle joint, and the talocalcaneal joint, which is usually referred to as the subtalar joint. The ankle joint consists of tibiotalar, fibulotalar and distal tibiofibular articulations. It resembles the mortise and tenon joint used in carpentry.

The talus is central to mechanics of foot and ankle, as it forms a series of joints that connect the foot to the leg:

- The body of the talus (talar dome) articulates in the ankle joint.
- The inferior aspect of the talus articulates in the subtalar joint.
- The head of the talus articulates in the talocalcanonavicular joint.

Through these articulations, the talus transmits the entire weight of the body to the foot. The talar dome has a wedge-shaped profile: it is wider at the front than at the back; it is also wider at the lateral aspect than at the medial aspect; furthermore, it is vertically longer at the lateral aspect than at the medial aspect. Therefore, the talus has the shape of a frustum of a cone.

Ankle dorsiflexion–plantarflexion arc

The main arc of motion of the ankle joint is dorsiflexion and plantarflexion in the sagittal plane. Normal walking requires a motion between 10° dorsiflexion and 15° plantarflexion, with a total motion of 25°. Ascending stairs requires 37° and descending stairs requires 56° of ankle motion.

The difference in the size of the medial and lateral aspects of the talar dome means that, during dorsiflexion, the talus also externally rotates 5° and slides backwards in the joint – these motions are reversed during ankle plantarflexion. In addition, ankle dorsiflexion is coupled with eversion and plantarflexion with inversion of the subtalar joint.

Loads acting at the ankle joint

The forces acting at the ankle joint vary during the gait cycle. It is estimated that, during walking, the ankle joint reaction force reaches three times the total body weight in the stance phase and more than five times the total body weight at heel-off. The joint reaction force can be as high as 13 times total body weight during running and jumping. The tibiotalar articulation carries about 5/6 of the force and the fibulotalar articulation carries the remaining 1/6 of the force.

The contact area of the joint also changes during the gait cycle. During ankle dorsiflexion, the joint contact area moves from posterior to anterior, and vice versa during plantarflexion. The joint contact area is greatest, and the average stress is lowest, in dorsiflexion; this is reversed in plantarflexion. The fibula also moves 1–3 mm distally and rotates medially when the ankle joint is loaded.

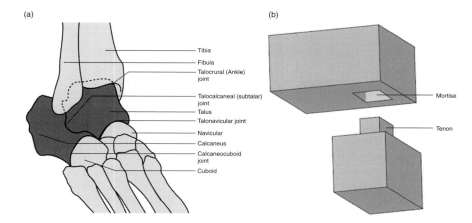

Fig. 11.1 The ankle is a unit of two joints: the talocrural joint, which is usually referred to as the ankle joint, and the talocalcaneal joint, which is usually referred to as the subtalar joint. The ankle joint resembles the mortise and tenon joint used in carpentry to join two pieces of wood together without glue or nails – the joint is stabilised by the congruency of the mating surfaces. The ankle joint is congruent through 96% of its dorsiflexion and plantarflexion arc. The supporting ligaments are also essential for joint stability.

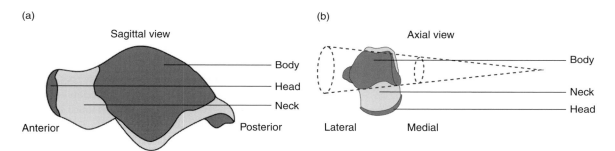

Fig. 11.2 The talus has the shape of a frustum of a cone. The asymmetry between the medial and lateral aspects allows the talus to rotate and slide within the joint during dorsiflexion and plantarflexion. Ankle dorsiflexion results in the wider anterior aspect of the talus engaging with the mortise, whereas ankle plantarflexion 'brings out' the talus and causes the narrower posterior aspect of the talus to engage within the mortise. Therefore, the ankle joint is close-packed and more stable in dorsiflexion, and is freer and less stable is plantarflexion (e.g. when wearing high-heeled shoes).

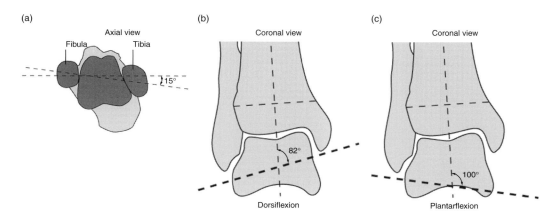

Fig. 11.3 The axis of motion of the ankle joint. (a) In the axial plane, the axis is angled posterolaterally. (b) In the coronal plane, the axis is angled inferolaterally in dorsiflexion, and (c) inferomedially during plantarflexion. Therefore, the ankle joint does not have a constant axis of motion, but instead has 'instant centres of rotation' that vary with joint position.

Total ankle replacement

Total ankle replacement is an alternative to arthrodesis for treatment of severe arthritis of the ankle.

Biomechanical considerations in total ankle replacement

The ankle joint presents unique biomechanical challenges for total ankle replacement:

- During the gait cycle, the ankle joint experiences large forces over a changing joint contact area. Therefore, stresses produced are non-uniformly distributed in the joint.
- The ligaments and other soft tissues surrounding the ankle joint are critical in maintaining the stability of the joint. These soft tissues also influence the distribution of stress in the joint.
- The articulating bones have a variable strength. The talus is almost one and half times stronger than the distal tibia, and the quality of both bones decreases significantly with the distance from the articular surface. Therefore, bone resection should ideally be less than 4 mm from the articular surface on each side, so that the resection surfaces can still support the prostheses under large compressive loads.

Design and alignment of components

The early total ankle replacement designs consisted mostly of two components: a polyethylene tibial component and a metal-based talar component. These components were fixed to the bone with cement. The bearing surfaces were either fully constrained or unconstrained; and both combinations produced very poor results.

Modern total ankle replacement designs consist of metal-based tibial and talar components with a polyethylene insert in the middle; the polyethylene insert is either fixed to the tibial or talar component or is 'mobile' between the surfaces. Most of the designs are cementless, with the components coated with hydroxyapatite to encourage bone growth on the prostheses for a stable bone–implant interface. Most designs also have a keel or a post at the back of the prostheses, which increases the bone–implant contact surface area and reduces pressure and micromotion between the surfaces. The cemented designs mostly have been abandoned because the use of cement requires much larger bone resections, due to the extra volume required to fit both the implants and the cement.

The bearing surfaces in a total ankle replacement need to be congruent to achieve as large a contact area as possible for load distribution, which increases joint stability and reduces wear of the polyethylene insert. However, bearing surfaces that are too congruent restrict the axial and translation motions required between the surfaces to increase the range of dorsiflexion–plantarflexion arc. Therefore, bearing surfaces in modern total ankle replacements achieve a balance between congruency and mobility.

Correct alignment of components is critical to prevent overloading of the joint. The most demanding step of the total ankle replacement operation is the correct positioning of the talar component. One of the most common complications after total ankle replacement is mal-position of the talar component in the sagittal plane (Table 11.1).

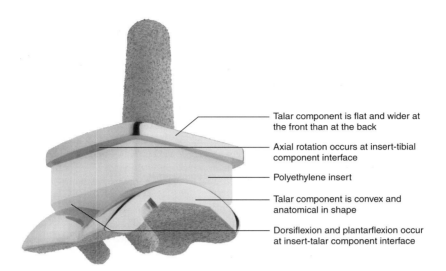

Talar component is flat and wider at the front than at the back

Axial rotation occurs at insert-tibial component interface

Polyethylene insert

Talar component is convex and anatomical in shape

Dorsiflexion and plantarflexion occur at insert-talar component interface

Fig. 11.4 Modern total ankle replacement designs consist of metal-based (usually cobalt–chrome) tibial and talar components and a polyethylene insert in the middle. In the example shown, the polyethylene insert is not fixed to the tibial insert and its motion is constrained only by friction and conformity with the opposing surfaces. The current total ankle replacement designs do not reproduce the convex–concave articulation of normal ankle joint, and therefore change the normal joint kinematics. (Image of Zenith™ Total Ankle Replacement – courtesy of Corin Group plc.)

Table 11.1. Clinical considerations in ankle arthrodesis and total ankle replacement

	Ankle arthrodesis	Total ankle replacement
Advantages	Ankle arthrodesis is a reliable pain-relieving procedure. At present, it is considered to be the surgical gold standard for end-stage ankle arthritis. It can be performed arthroscopically, which reduces the risk of complications and time to achieve joint fusion. Patients maintain a good level of activity after ankle fusion. It is durable, and recommended for patients who expect to continue with high-impact activity and workload.	Total ankle replacement restores joint range of motion. It is suitable for patients who do not expect to participate in vigorous activity. *Relative contraindications*: pre-operative ankle range of motion <20°, subtalar joint arthritis, poor condition of skin and soft tissues, laxity of collateral ligaments. *Absolute contraindications*: severe deformity of the joint, neuropathic joints and talar necrosis affecting >25% of talar dome.
Limitations and complications	Ankle arthrodesis does not restore range of motion. Therefore, patients may not be able to perform activities that require ankle movement, e.g. standing on tiptoe, jumping, squatting or lunging. Main complications are infection and painful non-union. There is also a risk of mal-union. Failure rate of ankle arthrodesis is between 5% and 10%. In the long term, it can also lead to arthritis in the adjacent subtalar joint, which can require subtalar joint fusion.	Total ankle replacement is a technically demanding procedure with a longer learning curve. Improvement in the ankle range of motion is typically between 0°–14°. It is unclear whether the increased motion actually leads to a better level of activity. Main complications are infection and aseptic loosening, with associated higher risk of major revision surgery. Survival rate of current designs at 5 years is between 67% and 94%, and at 10 years is 75%. Other complications include delay in wound healing and periprosthetic fractures, especially around the malleoli.

Three rockers of normal gait

The gait cycle describes how the musculoskeletal system achieves locomotion. The gait cycle extends from one heel-strike to the next heel-strike of the same leg. It consists of stance phase (65%) and swing phase (35%). The stance phase extends from heel-strike to toe-off on the same foot, and swing phase extends from toe-off to heel-strike on the same foot. In the stance phase, the leg is in contact with the ground and supports the body, whilst in the swing phase, it creates a new step forward.

In the stance phase, the mechanics of the foot and ankle is described in terms of three rockers.

- The first (heel) rocker is the very brief period between heel-strike and foot-flat, where the landing foot prepares to receive the load. The heel exerts a contact force on the ground and receives an equal and opposite ground reaction force. The point of application of ground reaction force is posterior to the ankle joint, which causes the ankle to move from neutral to 10° plantarflexion. The dorsiflexors of the ankle (mainly tibialis anterior) contract eccentrically to control the rate of this motion. Therefore, this is a deceleration rocker.
- The second (ankle) rocker is the much longer period between foot-flat and heel-off, where the firmly placed foot allows the supporting leg and the rest of the body to move forwards. Although the foot is on the ground, the change in relative position of the leg alters the ankle attitude from 10° plantarflexion to 10° dorsiflexion. The force for this change in ankle position is produced effectively by the point of application of the ground reaction force vector moving anterior to the ankle. The plantarflexors of the ankle (gastrocnemius and soleus) contract eccentrically to control the rate of ankle dorsiflexion. Therefore, this is also a deceleration rocker.
- The third (forefoot) rocker is the short period between heel-off and toe-off, where the supporting foot prepares to take off. The ankle position rapidly changes from 10° dorsiflexion to 20° plantarflexion. As the heel rises, the toes also undergo progressive extension, to a maximum just before toe-off. The ground reaction force vector is still acting anterior to the ankle joint, producing a dorsiflexion moment. However, the plantarflexors of the ankle contact concentrically to produce ankle plantarflexion. Therefore, this is an acceleration rocker.

In the swing phase, the leg is not in contact with the ground, and therefore does not experience a ground reaction force. The ankle dorsiflexors bring the ankle to a neutral position to permit toe clearance.

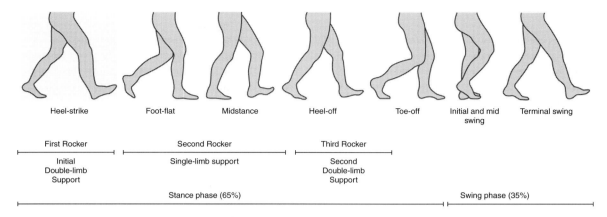

Heel-strike   Foot-flat   Midstance   Heel-off   Toe-off   Initial and mid   Terminal swing
                                                                swing

First Rocker   Second Rocker   Third Rocker

Initial   Single-limb support   Second
Double-limb   Double-limb
Support   Support

Stance phase (65%)   Swing phase (35%)

Fig. 11.5 The gait cycle extends from one heel-strike to the next heel-strike of the same leg.

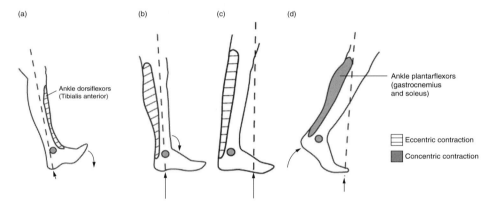

Fig. 11.6 The stance phase is divided into three rockers. The centre of gravity, and therefore the ground reaction force, moves forwards with each rocker. The muscles are contracting eccentrically in the first and second rockers and concentrically in the third rocker. An eccentric muscle contraction is in the opposite direction to the movement of the limb, i.e. the muscle lengthens as it contracts; a concentric muscle contraction is in the same direction as the movement of the limb, i.e. the muscle shortens as it contracts; and the isometric muscle contraction maintains the position of the limb, i.e. the muscle remains the same length as it contracts.

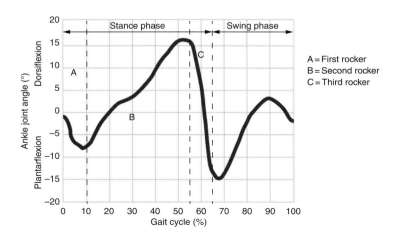

A = First rocker
B = Second rocker
C = Third rocker

Fig. 11.7 The ankle joint angle during the gait cycle. In the stance phase, the ankle briefly plantarflexes during the first rocker, dorsiflexes during the second rocker, and then rapidly plantarflexes during the third rocker. In the swing phase, the ankle comes back to the neutral position.

The foot

The foot has two main mechanical functions during walking: it acts as a shock absorber and mobile adaptor to adjust to uneven terrain; and as a rigid lever for forward propulsion. The foot functions in only one mode at any particular time. Each function is linked to a specific period of stance phase of the gait cycle: the foot acts a shock absorber and mobile adaptor during the first and second rockers and as a rigid lever during the third rocker. The subtalar joint is central to how the foot performs these contrasting functions, switching between them and timing them with the gait cycle.

The subtalar joint

The subtalar joint is the articulation between talus and calcaneus. The subtalar joint axis is half-way between the vertical axis of the leg and horizontal axis of the foot. This unique orientation of the subtalar joint allows it to function as what in engineering terms is described as a 'mitred hinge'. The subtalar joint can therefore convert rotation of the leg in the vertical plane to rotation of the foot in the horizontal plane. The foot rotation is produced in the transverse tarsal (midfoot) joints, i.e. the talonavicular and calcaneocuboidal joints, which are immediately adjacent to the subtalar joint.

Foot as a shock absorber and mobile adaptor

During the first rocker, the ankle joint plantarflexes (and rotates internally) briefly to bring down the foot. The soft tissues of the foot absorb energy in this period. The body has double-limb support for most of this time, so the foot has relatively low loads applied to it.

During the second rocker, the ankle joint dorsiflexes and rotates externally (i.e. the superimposed leg rotates internally). There is coupled eversion of the subtalar joint and the hind foot. The eversion of the subtalar joint rotates the transverse tarsal joints into congruent (parallel) alignment with each other. This makes the foot flexible and soft to absorb energy, as the single limb supports the body during this period.

Foot as a rigid lever

During the third rocker, the ankle joint plantarflexes and rotates internally (i.e. the superimposed leg rotates externally). There is coupled inversion of the subtalar joint and the hind foot. The inversion of the subtalar joint rotates the transverse tarsal joints into incongruent alignment with each other. This turns the foot into a rigid lever arm that can now be used for forward propulsion of the body.

In addition, as the heel rises, the toes also undergo progressive extension, to a maximum just before toe-off. The plantar fascia extends from the calcaneum to the base of the toes. Extension of the toes tightens the plantar fascia, which raises the foot arch and contributes to the rigid lever structure of the foot. This is known as the 'windlass' effect.

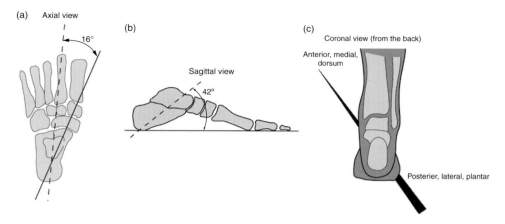

Fig. 11.8 The subtalar joint has an oblique axis in all three planes. The axis of the subtalar joint runs from a posterior, lateral, plantar position to an anterior, medial and dorsum position.

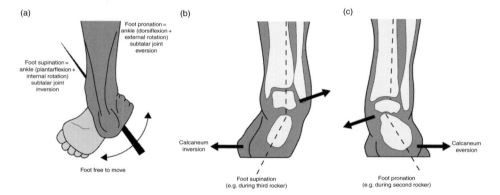

Fig. 11.9 Movement at the subtalar joint produces triplane motion. In addition, movements of the subtalar joints are *always* coupled with movements at the ankle joint. The observable effect of these coupled movements depends on whether (a) the foot is free or (b), (c) resting on the ground.

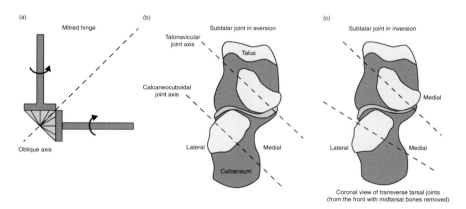

Fig. 11.10 The subtalar joint acts as a mitred hinge. (a) A mitred hinge has an oblique axis and acts as a torque convertor. During the second rocker, the leg rotates internally, the ankle dorsiflexes, the subtalar joint everts and the transverse tarsal joints become congruent (unlocked). This makes the foot flexible and soft. During the third rocker, the leg rotates externally, the ankle plantarflexes, the subtalar joint inverts and the transverse tarsal joints become incongruent (locked). This makes the foot a rigid lever.

Introduction to fracture fixation

The principles of fracture fixation are as follows:

1. Reduce the fracture

This can be achieved by: indirect method (i.e. closed reduction), which does not require exposure of the fracture; or direct method (i.e. open reduction), which involves formal exposure of the fracture. A fracture can also be reduced by a percutaneous method, which involves a limited direct access to the fracture to aid closed reduction.

Intra-articular fractures ideally require 'anatomic' reduction, to restore the articular surface. In contrast, extra-articular fractures usually only require 'adequate' (i.e. non-anatomical) reduction, as the goal is to restore the length, rotation and alignment of the bone, which usually does not require perfect reduction of the fracture.

2. Hold the fracture reduced until it is united

This can be achieved by external fixation or by internal fixation methods. The fracture does not heal any quicker whether treated by one method or the other. However, different fixation methods have different mechanisms for maintaining fracture reduction; some methods permit closed/adequate reduction, whilst other methods enable open/anatomic reduction. A fixation device is redundant once the fracture has healed.

3. Rehabilitation

This helps to reduce tissue oedema, preserve joint motion, improve muscle power and restore normal function of the limb. Internal fixation provides immediate skeletal stability and generally permits early rehabilitation and return to function.

It is useful to consider the different fracture fixation methods in terms of stiffness of the device and stability of the bone–device construct:

- *Stiffness* is the ability of a device to resist its deformation. It is also referred to as the rigidity of the device, and depends on the material and geometric properties of the device.
- *Stability* is the ability of the bone–device construct as a whole to maintain fracture reduction. The fracture and the device both contribute to stability. If the fracture provides less stability to the construct, the fixation device has to provide more.

The distinction between stiffness and stability is important because a device with low stiffness can still provide high fracture stability, and vice versa; stability is dependent on fracture configuration and reduction and on how the fixation device is applied. This is why, although a plate is usually less stiff than an intramedullary nail, plate fixation usually provides absolute stability, whereas an intramedullary nail fixation usually provides relative stability. In clinical practice, stability is often implied in term of the stiffness/rigidity of the bone–device construct. Therefore, this chapter refers to both the stability and stiffness of the bone–device construct (Tables 12.1 and 12.2).

Table 12.1. **Absolute stability vs relative stability**

The term 'absolute stability' implies maximum fracture stability with minimal relative motion between fracture fragments. Absolute stability is essential for primary bone healing, which is typically required in intra-articular fractures. Therefore, the principle of fixing intra-articular fractures is 'anatomic reduction, absolute stability'. The term 'relative stability' implies that there is some relative motion between fracture fragments. Relative stability is usually adequate for extra-articular fractures. Therefore, the principle of extra-articular fracture fixation is 'adequate reduction, relative stability'.

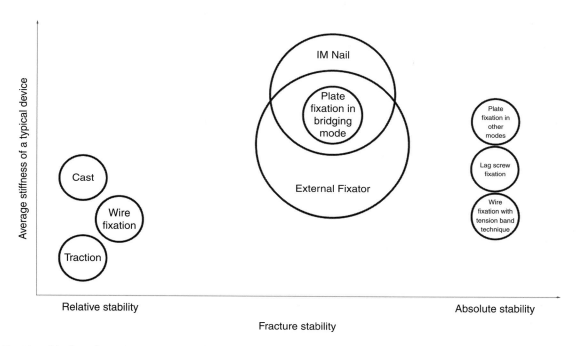

Fig. 12.1 This chart shows the spectrum of stiffness and stability in fracture fixation techniques. The stiffness of a device can be modified to meet the stability requirement of the fracture.

Table 12.2. **Load-bearing vs load-sharing device**

Load-sharing and load-bearing are commonly used terms in clinical practice. These are used to make a distinction between fixation devices based on distribution of load between bone and device. A load-bearing device carries most of the load applied to the bone–device construct and may lead to localised bone resorption and osteopenia due to stress-shielding effect. On the other hand, a load-sharing device leads to a more equal distribution of load. Conventionally, plates are considered to be load-bearing implants. However, any transient osteopenia associated with plate fixation is more likely to be due to associated vascular compromise from its application rather than from its load-bearing properties. On the other hand, intramedullary nails are considered to be load-sharing devices as these readily permit axial loading of the fracture.

BIOMECHANICS OF FRACTURE FIXATION

Traction I

Traction is the method of realigning a fractured bone by applying a tensile force to the affected limb. It works on the principle of ligamentotaxis, whereby a longitudinally applied tensile force causes the intact soft tissues surrounding the fracture, such as periosteum, ligaments and joint capsule, to guide the fracture fragments back together. The function of the applied force is to maintain tension in the soft tissues.

Traction is usually applied to reduce and stabilise fractures temporarily whilst awaiting definitive fixation. It is widely used in the lower limb, mainly for femoral fractures as well as for acetabular and tibial fractures. It can also be used as a long-term treatment in cases where an invasive surgical treatment cannot be performed e.g. when a patient is unfit for surgery. Traction is more commonly used as a long-term treatment in children. There are two main reasons for this: children have a greater potential for bone remodelling even if traction does not align the bones perfectly, and fracture healing time is much shorter in children than in adults.

Traction can be applied to the limb by a tie secured to the skin (skin traction) or connected to a metal pin fixed into the bone (skeletal traction). The tensile force is produced by attaching a weight to the other end of the tie, or by securing the tie to a fixed post and using the weight of the body as a distracting force. When a weight is used to produce the tensile force, it is common to include a pulley (or multiple pulleys) in the construct.

The load that can be applied with skin traction is limited by skin and soft tissues concerns, such as: risk of friction blisters; skin necrosis over bony prominences; and constriction leading to nerve palsy, tissue oedema or vascular complications. Therefore, skin traction may not reduce a fracture completely, but is usually adequate to provide pain relief and maintain alignment. Skin traction may need to be readjusted periodically to prevent slacking. Skin traction typically is used in the following cases: in children; when only a small load (<5 kg) is required to maintain fracture reduction; or, when it is required for the short term (a few days) only. Otherwise, it is more appropriate to apply skeletal traction. Skeletal traction may also be required if the conditions of the soft tissues do not permit application of skin traction, e.g. skin lacerations. The usual sites for insertion of the pins for skeletal traction in the lower limb are: distal femur and proximal tibia for femoral fractures; and calcaneum for tibial fractures. For a femoral fracture, a load of up to 10% of body weight can safely be applied through skeletal traction (Table 12.3).

(a)   (b)

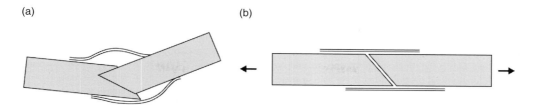

Fig. 12.2 Ligamentotaxis is the technique of reducing and stabilising a fracture by applying tension across the fracture using the intact soft tissues.

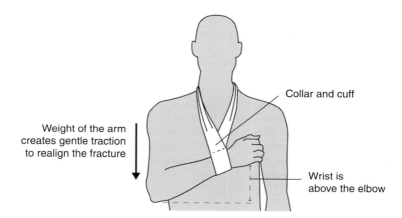

Fig. 12.3 Traction by gravity is used routinely for conservative management of proximal humerus fractures. The collar and cuff support the wrist above the elbow, and the weight of the unsupported arm creates a gentle traction that realigns the fracture. The arm can be taken out of the support for physiotherapy and personal care.

Table 12.3. **Traction: clinical perspective**

Traction is commonly used to achieve fracture reduction in a number of treatments. Manual traction is used to 'dis-impact' the fracture fragments during closed reduction of fractures, such as with an ankle or distal radial fracture. The surgeon usually requires the help of an assistant to apply manual traction; the surgeon applies traction to the limb on one side of the fracture, whilst the assistant stabilises the limb by applying 'counter-traction' on the opposite side of the fracture. Manual traction is also used for closed reduction of joint dislocations.

Traction is also used routinely in theatre to temporarily stabilise a fracture during a definitive fixation procedure. In this setting, traction can be achieved manually or by using special equipment, e.g. a traction table or a Chinese finger trap.

An external fixator also relies on traction (which in this context is also referred to as distraction) and the principle of ligamentotaxis to stabilise a fracture.

Traction by gravity is utilised for reducing certain fractures (and dislocations). The principle of traction by gravity is to place the limb in a gravity-dependent position so that the weight of the limb provides the traction.

Traction II

Traction is commonly used to stabilise femoral fractures. The following are the most common set-ups of traction for femoral fractures:

- *Straight traction*: This is the simplest type of traction, and can be used for femoral fracture in any age group. It involves application of longitudinal traction using either skin or skeletal traction.
- *Thomas splint*: This is a portable traction splint that provides straight traction to the fractured femur. It involves application of skin traction to the injured leg by placing it in an appropriate size splint. The tie of the skin traction is secured to the distal end of the splint to provide a traction force. The Thomas splint is used routinely in the pre-hospital setting to transfer patients with femoral fractures. It may also be used with additional equipment, e.g. additional ties and pulleys, to provide long-term conservative treatment of the fracture.
- *Gallow's traction*: This is used for an infant with a femoral fracture. Both the fractured and the uninjured leg are placed in skin traction and suspended in air from an overhead frame. The hips are flexed to 90° and the legs are pulled vertically upwards. The correct amount of traction allows the buttocks to only slightly lift off the bed (to allow change of nappy). The child's weight provides counter-traction to splint the fracture. This traction method can be used for infants up to about 12 kg or 18 months of age.
- *The 90°–90° traction*: This is used typically in an older child with a subtrochanteric fracture of the femur, where the proximal fragment tends to flex and abduct due to the action of the attached psoas and gluteal muscles. The hip and knee are both flexed to 90°, which relaxes the muscles acting on the femur. In addition, an upwards force is applied to the distal fragment to stabilise the fracture. This usually needs to be applied through skeletal traction.
- *Balanced (Hamilton–Russell) traction*: This involves application of two perpendicular forces to the leg, which is slightly flexed at the knee: an upwards force and a longitudinal force. The resultant vector of the two forces is a tensile force that acts in line with the femur. Balanced traction can also be used to control the rotation of the leg, by directing the upwards force medially or laterally. Generally, the limb has the tendency to rotate externally in traction, and the upwards force can be adjusted to ensure that the patella is pointing directly upwards.

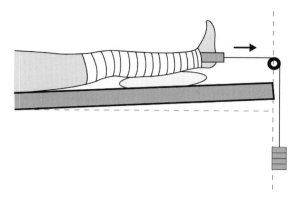

Fig. 12.4 Straight traction: this example shows the use of the skin traction technique to apply longitudinal traction to the limb. The padding under the leg prevents the heel from pressing into the bed, which could cause pressure sores. The end of the bed is raised slightly to prevent the patient from slipping down.

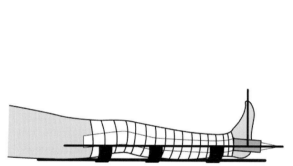

Fig. 12.5 A Thomas splint combines skin traction with a portable frame.

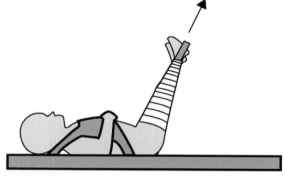

Fig. 12.6 Gallow's traction is used for an infant with a femoral fracture. It may be continued until the fracture unites or is converted to a hip spica cast during the treatment.

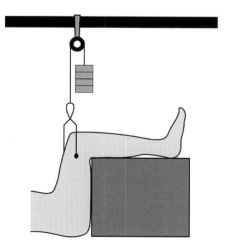

Fig. 12.7 The 90°–90° traction involves flexing the hip and knee to 90°. This can be achieved by raising the leg on a support or by applying a sling under the calf and suspending it from the frame.

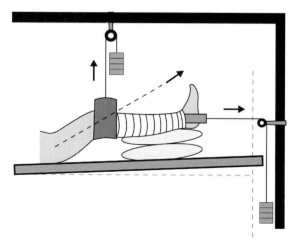

Fig. 12.8 Balanced traction involves application of an upwards and a longitudinal force to the leg. The leg is slightly flexed at the knee. The resultant vector of the two forces is a tensile force that acts in the line of the femur.

Cast

A cast is a non-invasive external splint used to stabilise fractures. It can be used in combination with other fixation methods to provide additional support.

Biomechanics of cast

The two most commonly used materials with which to make casts are plaster of Paris and fibreglass, although plastic and metal are also used routinely. Plaster of Paris is weak in tension and much stronger in compression, and so is prone to break down in regions under tension. Fibreglass is a lighter, stiffer and stronger material than plaster of Paris. In addition, unlike plaster of Paris, fibreglass is water resistant. However, as fibreglass is stiffer, its casts are less accommodating of soft tissue swelling and are more difficult to mould, which can result in formation of sharp edges. The stiffness of cast made from both materials increases with the number of layers used (i.e. thickness of the cast).

Biomechanics of bone–cast construct

Different types of casts are used for treating different fractures, and the stability of bone–cast construct depends on the bone fractured, the fracture pattern and the form of cast. There are four main groups of cast:

- *Back slab*: This is a splint that only partly encircles the limb. It is usually applied in the acute setting to stabilise the fracture temporarily, whilst accommodating soft tissue swelling.
- *Full cast*: This encircles the full circumference of the limb. In principle, the joint above and the joint below the fracture are usually also immobilised with the full cast to increase stability of the construct and therefore reduce the risk of fracture displacement.
- *Spica*: This encircles a part of the body, e.g. hip spica and thumb spica.
- *Functional brace*: This encircles the full circumference of the limb, but does not impede motion of the adjacent joint. A functional brace may be developed from a range of materials. The mechanics of a functional brace are considered on pages 193–194.

It is essential that the first three types of cast be moulded to provide three-point fixation of the fracture, which increases construct stability. The traditional orthopaedic saying is that 'a straight (unmoulded) cast leads to bent bones (i.e. loss of fracture reduction) and a bent (moulded) cast leads to straight bones'. Three-point fixation is provided by a combination of mechanisms:

- direct buttressing effect of the moulded cast on the fracture fragments
- principle of ligamentotaxis – provided by the 'soft tissue hinge' around the fracture
- hydraulic compression forces of the muscles surrounding the fracture.

It is also important that a cast is of adequate length to obtain proper fracture stabilisation.

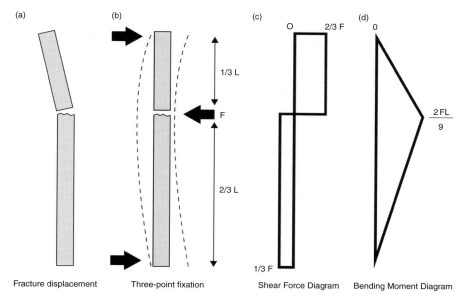

Fig. 12.9 A fracture often requires closed reduction before application of a cast. (a) An angulated fracture, e.g. of distal radius, is reduced by applying a force opposite to the initial deforming force. (b) The fracture is stabilised with three-point fixation applied by a moulded full cast. The stabilised bone may be considered as a beam subjected to three-point loading (see pages 54–55). The geometry of the forces determines the loads applied to each bone fragment. An important inference from this analysis is that the shear force acts uniformly along the entire length of a bone fragment involved in three-point fixation up to the point of application of the next force (c), (d).

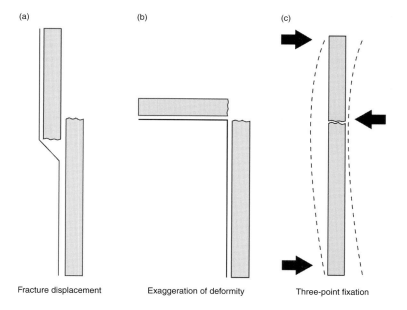

Fig. 12.10 Reduction of an off-ended fracture may require exaggeration of deformity as part of the reduction technique. (a) The off-ended fracture usually has an intact soft tissue hinge on the side that the distal fragment has translated to, and ruptured soft tissues on the opposite side. Simple traction or a bending force may not be sufficient to reduce the fracture. (b) Therefore, fracture deformity needs to be increased to approximate the opposing ends of the fracture, after which (c) the fracture can be reduced and three-point fixation applied. This technique is particularly important in children, in whom the periosteum is thick and resilient.

Wires

Wires have a wide array of uses in fracture fixation. Wires are typically made from stainless steel and are available in a range of sizes and finishes.

Biomechanics of wires

A wire's stiffness is proportional to its radius to the fourth power. Wires generally are relatively flexible and can be easily bent. Wires can be broadly divided into two types:

- *Kirschner (k)-wires*: These are relatively stiff, straight wires with sharp, pointed tips. However, there are many variations to this basic design.
- *Cerclage wires*: These flexible wires often come in a coil, and can be wound around fracture fragments to reduce and hold them in position.

Biomechanics of bone–wire construct

Fracture fixation with k-wires

The following are important considerations in fracture fixation with k-wires.

- The fracture should be reduced satisfactorily. A wire can sometimes be used to 'lever' a fragment into position.
- The diameter of a wire should be appropriate for the size of the bone and fracture fragments.
- Construct stability increases with the number of wires fixing the fracture, but two to three wires are optimal for most fractures.
- If multiple wires are used, they must not cross each other at the fracture site, as this may splint the fracture apart.
- In most cases, a wire should ideally 'bite' the far cortex to prevent backing out.
- In most cases, the fixation requires further stabilisation with a plaster or splint until the fracture is sufficiently united for the wires to be removed. The fracture typically heals with callus formation.

Tension band principle

This is a classical engineering concept. Principles of tension band wire fixation are as follows:

- It is typically applied to bones that are eccentrically loaded, e.g. for olecranon and patella fractures. A cerclage wire band applied to the tension side of a fracture neutralises the distracting force and can even convert it into a uniform compressive force.
- Fractures suitable for tension band wire are typically transverse or short oblique with no significant comminution at the far cortex.
- The fracture is reduced anatomically and usually two parallel k-wires are also passed across the fracture to act as rails along which the fragments compress. k-Wires should ideally cross the fracture close to the far cortex for maximum mechanical leverage.
- The fracture typically unites by primary bone healing, which is the goal since most fractures requiring tension band fixation are intra-articular.

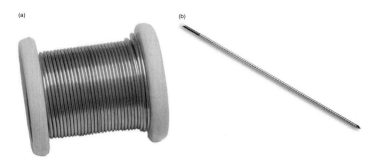

Fig. 12.11 There are two groups of wires: k-wires and cerclage wires. Thicker wires are conventionally referred to as pins; a wire is usually between 0.9 and 1.5 mm in diameter, whereas a pin is usually between 1.5 and 6.5 mm in diameter. (Image (a) is reproduced with permission of Narang Medial Ltd. Image (b) is reproduced with permission of Disposable Instrument Co.)

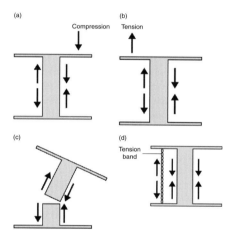

Fig. 12.12 Tension band principle. A structure acts as a beam when subjected to eccentric loading – the load can be compressive or tensile. If there is a break in the continuity of the structure, the eccentric load causes it to rotate as well as translate. A band applied to the tensile surface takes up the tensile component of the load, thereby allowing stabilising compressive component to act on the structure. Wires are the most common means of achieving tension band effect, but sutures, screws and plates can also be used to produce this effect. The tension band principle is less effective when there is significant comminution of the fracture, especially at a compressive surface.

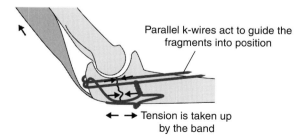

Fig. 12.13 Tension band wire fixation of olecranon fracture. This can also be applied to fractures of the patella, medial malleolus of the ankle and tuberosities of the proximal humerus.

Surgical screw I

The screw is a simple machine that converts a torque into an axial force. The screw is commonly used to hold materials together for assembly and construction, although the 'screw thread mechanism' has a variety of applications, e.g. corkscrew, screw top container lid and the Archimedes' screw to move materials. A surgical screw may be made of metal, e.g. stainless steel or titanium, or a biodegradable material, e.g. biodegradable polymers.

Biomechanics of screw

The screw thread mechanism converts rotational motion into linear motion. The torque applied to the screw head turns the cylindrical shaft and the outer helical threads. The helix couples rotational motion to linear motion. The linear motion in turn generates axial force. Importantly, an axial force applied to the screw shaft cannot make the screw turn back the other way.

Although there are many different designs of screw, the basic mechanical properties of any screw are determined by the following key characteristics:

- *Head*: This permits attachment of the screwdriver and halts screw advancement into a material. The coupling interface for the screwdriver is typically hexagonal or star shaped. This design prevents the screwdriver from losing grip, whilst spreading the stress from the screwdriver over a large surface area. The under-surface of the screw head is usually round to also maximise the area over which the stress from the screw head is spread across the underlying surface.
- *Neck*: This is the section between the screw head and threads. It is usually the weakest section of the screw, and where a screw usually breaks. A fully threaded screw has a very short neck, whereas a partially threaded screw has a longer neck.
- *Core diameter*: This is the diameter of the cylindrical shaft. It determines the stiffness of the screw and its resistance to fatigue failure. It also determines the diameter of the drill that should be used to create the hole for the screw.
- *Outer diameter*: This is the diameter of the screw threads. This is also the minimum hole diameter through which the screw will glide without its threads engaging. A surgical screw is usually referred to by this diameter, e.g. a 3.5 mm cortical screw has a thread diameter of 3.5 mm.
- *Pitch*: This is the distance between screw threads. It corresponds to the linear distance a screw travels for each complete turn. The screw amplifies a small torque into a large axial force; the force amplification effect is inversely proportional to the pitch. In other words, the smaller the linear distance a screw travels for each complete turn (i.e. output distance < input distance), the greater the axial force produced for a given torque (i.e. output force > input force) – this is due to the force–distance relationship in simple machines, which is explained on pages 12–13 (Table 12.4).

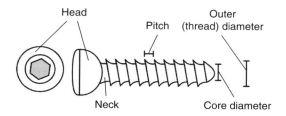

Fig. 12.14 The functional anatomy of a screw. The screw's hold in the bone is referred to as purchase. The axial force required to remove a screw is referred to as its pullout strength. The pullout strength of a screw can be increased by increasing the contact surface area (interference) between screw threads and bone. This can be achieved by increasing the outer diameter or reducing the core diameter (which effectively increases width of the threads) or the pitch.

Table 12.4. **The different types of surgical screws**

Surgical screws come as fully or partially threaded. A fully threaded screw has threads along its whole length, whereas a partially threaded screw has threads only part-way along from the screw tip.

A screw designed to gain purchase mainly in the cortices of the bone is referred to as a cortical screw. Similarly, a screw designed to gain purchase mainly in the cancellous bone is referred to as a cancellous screw. The cortical bone is usually dense but has limited thickness, whereas cancellous bone is much less dense and more spread out. Therefore, to maximise purchase, cortical screws have a small pitch and their tips are designed to cut into dense cortical bone, whereas cancellous screws have wider threads and larger pitch and their tips are designed to press cancellous bone aside, much like a snow plough presses aside spread-out snow.

A self-tapping screw has a cutting flute at the tip, which cuts a channel into the bone for screw threads. It can be inserted directly after a hole is drilled into the bone. A screw that is not self-tapping has a plain tip and requires the drilled hole to be separately tapped before it can be applied.

A standard screw has a solid central core, whereas a cannulated screw has a canal through the central core, which can be used to guide the screw over a guide wire. A cannulated screw has a bigger core diameter than a standard screw of similar size. This maintains the stiffness of the screw, but since the threads' span is reduced, the cannulated screw has a lower pullout strength.

A locking screw is a special type of screw that has an additional set of threads around the head. It is used in combination with a 'locking' plate, which has reciprocal grooves around the plate holes. The locking screw therefore locks into the plate. This makes the plate–screw construct much more rigid than a non-locking construct, which provides greater stability to fixation.

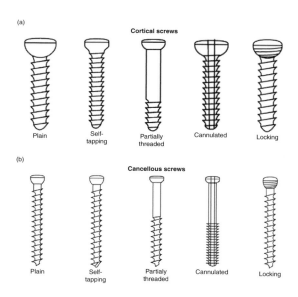

Fig. 12.15 Examples of the different types of surgical screws. (a) Cortical screws. (b) Cancellous screws. Left to right show the following properties in each set: plain, self-tapping, partially threaded, cannulated and locking. A screw may have different combinations of these properties, e.g. a cortical screw may be locking, self-tapping and cannulated.

Surgical screw II

Biomechanics of a bone–screw construct

A surgical screw can be used to hold bone fragments together or to affix an implant, e.g. plate, to the bone.

Fracture fixation with lag screw

A lag screw is used to affix bone fragments together – 'lag' is the mode in which a screw is applied, rather than a specific type of screw. Therefore, in principle any screw can function as a lag screw. The lag screw is applied after the fracture has been reduced anatomically. It can be applied independently or through a plate hole.

   Fully and partially threaded screws are applied as a lag screw using different techniques.

   A fully threaded screw achieves inter-fragmentary compression when applied using the lag technique.
- The lag technique is most effective in oblique fractures that are approximately twice as long as the bone diameter.
- As before, it is essential that the screw is applied perpendicular to the fracture line.
- The near fragment is over-drilled to the size of the outer diameter of screw (glide hole).
- The far fragment is drilled to the same size as the core diameter of the screw (pilot hole).
- The cortex of near fragment is 'countersunk', so that stress from the screw head is distributed over a large surface area.
- As the screw is applied, its threads engage in the far fragment but not in the near fragment.
- With further tightening, the screw head contacts the cortex of the near fragment and compresses it against the far fragment.
- Fully threaded screws are typically used in diaphyseal fractures, where the cortex is thick.

A partially threaded screw automatically achieves inter-fragmentary compression due to its design.
- As before, it is essential that the screw is applied perpendicular to the fracture line.
- The near and far fragments are drilled to the same size as the core diameter of the screw.
- As the screw is applied, the screw threads engage in the far fragment, but the unthreaded proximal section of the screw does not engage in the near fragment. It is therefore essential that all the screw threads are beyond the fracture and that no threads are in the near fragment or across the fracture.
- With further tightening, the screw head contacts the cortex of the near fragment and compresses it against the far fragment.
- Partially threaded screws are typically used in metaphyseal fractures, where the cortex is thin. Here, a washer may also be used under the screw head to prevent the screw head from being pushed through the cortex.
- Partially threaded screws are always applied as a lag screw.
- Most of the partially threaded screws used in fracture management are cancellous screws, and partially threaded cortical screws are not commonly used.

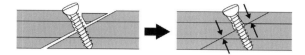

Fig. 12.16 Lag screw by technique: a fully threaded cortical screw acts as a lag screw when applied using the lag technique. It is essential that the screw is applied perpendicular to the fracture line. More than one screw can be applied, depending on the fracture pattern, fracture length and bone quality. A lag screw is usually not adequate to resist shear and torsional forces whilst the fracture heals. Therefore, it is usually also necessary to protect the lag screw fixation. In the small bones, e.g. in the hand, a second screw is applied across the fracture with the same technique as before except that the screw is applied perpendicular to the long axis of the bone. This is a 'neutralising' screw, as this is the optimal position for resisting shear forces. In larger bones, a neutralising plate is required to protect the lag screw fixation.

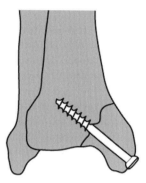

Fig. 12.17 Lag screw by design: a partially threaded cancellous screw automatically functions as a lag screw. This example shows fixation of a medial malleolar fracture of the ankle.

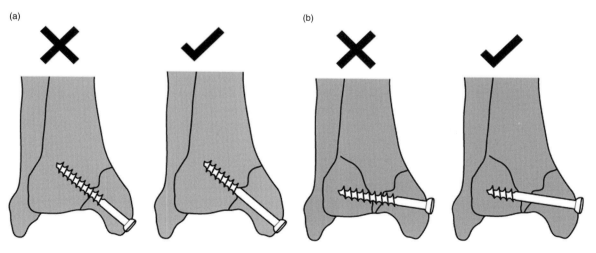

Fig. 12.18 In order for the partially threaded cancellous screws to achieve inter-fragmentary compression, it is essential that all the screw threads are beyond the fracture and that no threads are in the near fragment or across the fracture.

Plate fixation I

Plates are the most ubiquitous of fracture fixation implants. Plates are available in a variety of sizes and designs, and can be applied in a number of different modes.

Biomechanics of plate

The plate has the structure of a rectangular beam. Therefore, its stiffness is proportional to its width, and to its thickness to the third power. Changing the thickness of a plate has a greater effect on its stiffness than changing the base material.

Biomechanics of bone–plate construct I

Conventional plate vs locking plate

The conventional plate relies on friction between plate and bone for construct stability. This inevitably leads to compromise in the periosteal blood supply. The screws affix plate to bone, and also rely on friction to maintain hold in the bone. The quality of fixation is therefore limited by the bone quality. The screws are prone to a 'toggle' effect, i.e. the screws can rotate away from the applied position, and can also pull out on their own, which can weaken the fixation.

The locking plate has threaded holes, which allow the screw heads to lock into the plate. The locked screws are fixed in their position, which prevents them from toggling and backing out of the plate. The screws and the locking plate together form a 'fixed-angle' appliance, which is inherently much more stable than a non-locking interface between plate and screws. The bone–plate contact is not critical, and the periosteal blood supply is preserved. The plate therefore acts as an 'internal' external fixator. Fracture fixation with a locking plate is particularly desirable when there is less support provided by the bone, e.g. when bone quality is poor, as in osteoporosis, or if there is extensive fracture comminution.

Stiffness of bone–plate construct

The stiffness of bone–plate construct increases with the number of screws stabilising the bone fragments. The construct stiffness is also influenced by the distance between the screws closest to the fracture on either side; these screws experience the most force and construct stiffness decreases as the distance between them increases.

The stiffness of bone–plate construct also varies with the direction of loading. This is because the plate has different cross-sectional properties in different planes. Therefore, the construct's stiffness is determined by the plate's orientation to the plane of loading. Based on this concept, double-plate fixation of a fracture creates an even stiffer construct. Although the two plates can be applied in any arrangement, orthogonal plating, i.e. two plates applied at 90° degrees to each other, in principle improves construct stiffness uniformly in all planes. However, modern plates and fracture fixation techniques mean that most fractures do not routinely require double-plate fixation. Elbow supracondylar fractures and tibial pilon fractures are examples of where double-plate fixation is still used routinely.

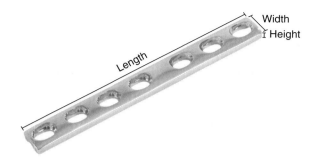

Fig. 12.19 The stiffness of a plate is proportional to its width, and to its thickness to the third power. A small increase in the thickness of the plate greatly increases its stiffness. (Reproduced with permission of Panchal Meditech.)

(a)

(b)

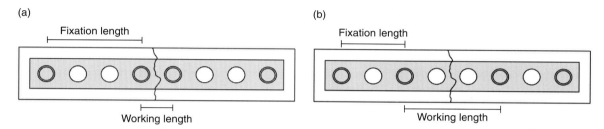

Fig. 12.20 The stiffness of bone–plate construct is influenced by the distance between the screws closest to the fracture on either side. This is also referred to as the working length of the plate. There is an inverse relationship between working length and fixation length. The stiffness of the construct decreases as the working length increases.

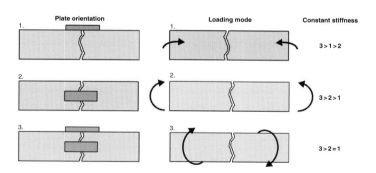

Fig. 12.21 The stiffness of bone–plate construct depends on the orientation of the plate to the plane of loading.

Plate fixation II

Biomechanics of bone–plate construct II

Modes of application

A plate can be used in a number of different modes, based on fracture location and pattern and the type of fracture stability required:

Neutralisation   Lag screws produce excellent inter-fragmentary compression, but are often inadequate to resist fracture displacement under functional loads. A plate can be applied across the fracture to provide further stiffness to the construct. The plate therefore 'neutralises' the forces and protects lag screw fixation from failure. A lag screw can also be applied through the plate hole, in which case it affixes the plate to the bone and compresses the fracture.

Compression   A plate can be applied to produce compression across a fracture. This is achieved by applying the first screw in a neutral position in a plate hole on one side of the fracture and then by applying the second screw in an eccentric position in a plate hole on the other side of the fracture. This screw configuration pulls the fragments together, producing inter-fragmentary compression. This technique can be used up to twice if required, but the first eccentric screw needs to be slightly loosened just before tightening the second eccentric screw to permit movement of fragments, after which it is tightened up again. Further screws can then be inserted as normal.

Bridging   It is not always necessary to fix every fragment in a multi-fragmentary fracture. A plate can be applied across a comminuted fracture and fixed to the bone at intervals. The aims of a bridging plate are to: minimise soft tissue disruption at the fracture zone and therefore preserve fracture blood supply; and splint the fracture in correct length, rotation and alignment. A plate applied in bridging mode is at an increased risk of fatigue failure because the bone–plate construct is likely to be less stable than in other modes due to fracture characteristics, e.g. comminution, bone loss or poor-quality bone, which may also lead to impaired bone healing.

Buttress/Antiglide   The term buttress means to support or reinforce. A plate is applied in buttress mode when a fracture has an apex/axilla; a plate applied to this surface of the fracture prevents sliding motion between fragments. The plate therefore resists shear forces between fragments. A buttress plate supports an intra-articular fracture and an antiglide plate supports a diaphyseal fracture – both modes work on the same principle.

Tension band   Most long bones in the body are loaded eccentrically, so that the adjacent sides of the bones are in tension and compression. A plate applied to the tension side of the bone neutralises tensile force and can even produce compression at the fracture site simply due to the tension band effect, i.e. when the tension side of a bone is splinted (banded), eccentric loading leads to fracture compression (this is further discussed on pages 166–177).

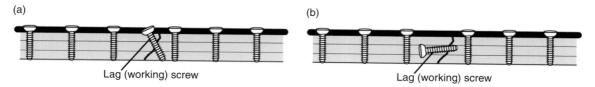

(a)

(b)

Lag (working) screw

Lag (working) screw

Fig. 12.22 Neutralisation mode. Primary fracture fixation is provided by the lag screw. The function of the plate is to neutralise (withstand) the applied load and protect lag screw fixation. The lag screw may be applied through the plate or independently of it. A lag screw is often also referred to as the 'working' screw, to distinguish it from the 'holding' screws in the plate.

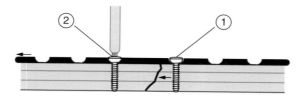

② ①

Fig. 12.23 Compression mode. The plate provides compression across the fracture. This is achieved through a specific method of screw placement. The first screw is inserted as normal. The second screw is inserted on the opposite side of the fracture and on the side of the plate hole away from the fracture. As the screw is inserted, the plate moves to accommodate the screw. The first screw has fixed the plate to the first bone fragment, which moves with the plate towards the fracture.

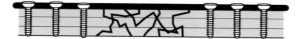

Fig. 12.24 Bridging mode. The plate acts as an extramedullary splint. It is usually inserted away from the fracture using minimally invasive technique and passed across the fracture without directly exposing it. The screws are inserted with short 'stab' incisions under fluoroscopy control. The bridging plate therefore allows the fracture to be stabilised with minimal disturbance to the soft tissue envelope around the fracture site. This is the only mode of plate application where the fracture is expected to heal by secondary bone healing with callous formation.

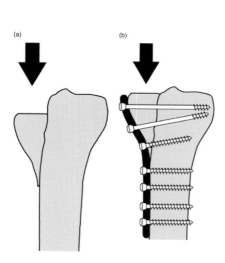

(a)

(b)

Fig. 12.25 Buttress/ Antiglide mode. The application of plate to the apex surface of the fracture inhibits shear motion between the fragments. A buttress plate supports an intra-articular fracture and an antiglide plate supports a diaphyseal fracture.

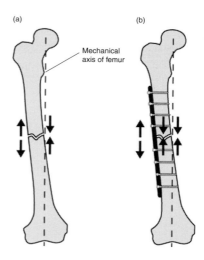

(a)

(b)

Mechanical axis of femur

Fig. 12.26 Tension band mode. Plate fixation can also achieve compression across the fracture by the way the bone is loaded. An eccentrically loaded bone, e.g. femur, acts like a beam with its one side under compression and the other under tension. A plate applied to the tensile surface takes up the tensile component of the load, and allows the stabilising compressive component to act at the fracture site.

Intramedullary nail I

An intramedullary (IM) nail acts as an internal splint to stabilise bone fragments. It is contoured typically to the profile of the bone.

Biomechanics of intramedullary nail

The IM nail is a cylindrical tube; therefore its stiffness is proportional to its radius to the fourth power. Therefore, a small increase in the radius has a big effect on the stiffness of the implant.

A solid nail is stiffer than a hollow nail of the same diameter. However, a hollow nail has a number of benefits.

- Less material is required to make a hollow nail than a solid nail. It is therefore also lighter.
- The central canal of the hollow nail can be used to guide the nail into position over a guide wire.

Hollow nails are therefore used routinely in the management of long bone fractures. The size of the central canal is carefully determined to limit the reduction in stiffness; although the outer radius of the nail has a far greater impact on stiffness than the thickness of the wall (see pages 56–57).

Biomechanics of bone–nail construct

Proximal and distal interlocking screws, referred to as 'bolts' in this role, provide rotational stability to the construct. Bolts are placed closer to the ends of the nail, which extends the zone of fractures that can be treated with a nail, but this is at the expense of construct stability. The rotational alignment of fragments is set when the first bolt is introduced into the second fragment after interlocking the first fragment. Bolts can be used in 'static' or 'dynamic' settings to control motion at the fracture.

The working length of the nail is the segment of nail around the fracture that is unsupported by bone. This is inversely related to construct stability:

- The nail is supported by bone where it is press-fixed to bone cortices, and the nail and bone both support the applied load. This is mainly in the diaphyseal region, where bone has the narrowest diameter, which therefore limits the maximum diameter of nail that can be used.
- The nail is not supported by bone at the fracture site, and the load is supported by the nail only. The nail is 'off-loaded' at the first point of contact between nail and bone on either side of the fracture – the distance between these two points is the working length of the nail.
- The working length of a nail press-fixed to the bone is determined by fracture pattern and location.
  - Transverse diaphyseal fractures lead to a working length of a few millimetres.
  - Comminuted diaphyseal fractures produce a longer working length.
  - In metaphyseal fractures, working length is between the bolt closest to the fracture and the first point of contact between nail and bone at the diaphysis.
- The working length of a nail with no surface contact with bone is between the bolts closest to the fracture on either side, regardless of fracture pattern and location.

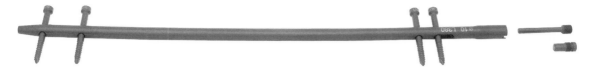

Fig. 12.27 The stiffness of an IM nail is proportional to its radius to the fourth power. Therefore, for the same wall thickness, a hollow nail with a 16 mm outer diameter is three times stiffer than one with an 11 mm outer diameter. Proximal and distal bolts provide rotational stability. IM nails are loosely referred to as IM rods. However, in mechanics, a rod is solid whereas a tube is hollow. Therefore, it is more appropriate to refer to a solid nail as an IM rod and a hollow nail as an IM tube. (Image courtesy of MEDIN.)

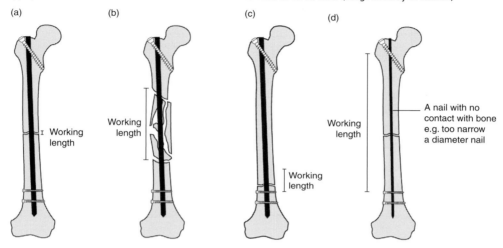

Fig. 12.28 The working length of nail is the segment of nail around the fracture that is unsupported by bone.

Applying conditions of equilibrium:

1. Sum of all moments is zero.

∴ taking moments about the fracture site:

Total clockwise moment = Total anticlockwise moment

$$F_{screw} \times D_{screw} = F_{Bone} \times D_{Bone}$$

$$\therefore F_{screw} = \frac{F_{Bone} \times D_{Bone}}{D_{Screw}}$$

since $D_{Bone} \gg D_{Screw}$

$$\therefore F_{Screw} \gg F_{Bone}$$

2. Sum of all forces is zero.

$$\therefore F = F_{Bone} + F_{Screw}$$

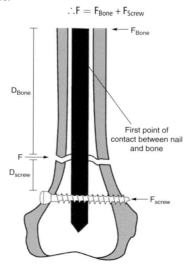

Fig. 12.29 External loads and muscles forces produce bending stress between IM nail and bone. The bending stresses are greatest at the fracture site. An IM nail fixation of a fracture of the distal third of a long bone generates high stresses on the adjacent interlocking bolts. This may lead to failure of these bolts.

Intramedullary nail II

Flexible IM nails are a subgroup of the IM nail family, and function with different biomechanical principles. A flexible IM nail combines elasticity and stability in one construct and is also referred to as an 'elastic stable IM nail'.

Biomechanics of a flexible IM nail

These are made from stainless steel or titanium. The stiffness of the nail is proportional to its radius to the fourth power.

Biomechanics of bone–nail construct

Flexible IM nails are used most commonly in the management of paediatric femoral and forearm bones fractures. These provide a number of surgical advantages over other fracture fixation methods. These are minimally invasive, relatively safe to insert and remove, present low risk of physeal injury and allow early mobilisation. The nails are usually removed after fracture union, and the risk of re-fracture is low.

Femoral fractures

The strain energy stored in the construct provides fixation stability:
- Two nails are applied retrograde to prevent injury to the proximal and distal femoral physes.
- Both nails have the same diameter, which ideally should be 40% of the internal diameter of the medullary canal at its narrowest (diaphysis).
- Both nails are bent together, and the apex of the bend lies at the fracture site.
- The nails are introduced from opposite cortices to form diametrically opposite curves at the fracture site.
- Each nail provides 'trifocal buttressing' (i.e. three-point fixation), to the fracture.
- The construct has excellent stability under axial and bending loads, but is still relatively weak under rotational load. It is stable enough for the patient to mobilise bearing partial weight on the limb.
- The fracture heals by secondary bone healing.
- Flexible IM nails are typically used to manage femoral fractures in children between the ages of 5 and 14 years with body weight up to 50 kg. They may be used in even older, heavier children, but additional protection, e.g. with a cast brace, may be required to maintain adequate stability.

Forearm bone fractures

Flexible IM nails are sometimes used to internally splint radius and ulna fractures:
- Generally, only unstable, displaced or open fractures require fixation. Therefore, if both bones are fractured, it is not always necessary to fix them both. If one fracture is displaced and the other is not, then fixing one fracture may provide adequate stability to the forearm as a unit.
- A single nail is used for each forearm bone, and is usually inserted anterograde in the ulna and retrograde in the radius.
- The diameter of the nail is determined by the size of the medullary canal of the bone and is usually between 2.0 and 2.5 mm.
- The construct requires additional protection with a cast.
- The fracture heals by secondary bone healing.

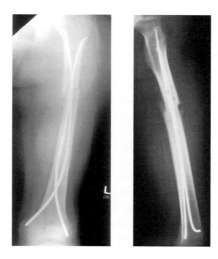

Fig. 12.30 These radiographs show an example of the use of flexible nails to stabilise a femoral fracture. Flexible nails are ideal for mid-diaphyseal fractures with a transverse, short oblique or short spiral pattern, although these may also be considered for more peripheral or multi-fragmented fractures in selected cases.

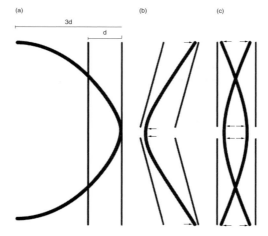

Fig. 12.31 Principles of elastic stability. The nails are bent (i.e. plastic deformation) so that the height of the apex of the curve is three times the diameter of the femoral diaphysis. As a pre-contoured nail is inserted into the relatively straight medullary canal, it is forced to straighten out (i.e. elastic deformation). This creates a bending moment that tends to angulate the fracture. This is balanced by the moment produced by the opposite nail.

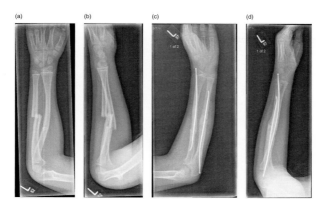

Fig. 12.32 These radiographs show an example of the application of flexible nails to stabilise radius and ulna fracture.

External fixation I

External fixation is a method of stabilising a fracture by applying implants to the bone that extend outside the soft tissues and are externally linked by an adjustable beam system. The components of an external fixator are away from the fracture environment. This is advantageous in situations such as open fractures with risk of infection and in fractures associated with massive soft tissue injury where the external fixation does not disturb the zone of injury.

External fixators may be used for temporary or definitive fracture stabilisation, and are divided into pin-to-bar, ring or hybrid types. Pin-to-bar fixators are applied in routine trauma surgery, e.g. open fractures, peri-articular injury and polytrauma, whereas ring fixators are usually applied in more complex reconstruction situations, e.g. fracture mal-union or non-union, bone infection and limb deformity correction. Temporarily applied external fixators are converted to definitive internal fixation when the fracture environment is suitable.

As an external fixator consists of different units, its rigidity depends on the properties of its components and their spatial configuration. An external fixator provides 'flexible' stiffness to the healing fracture because its components and their arrangement can be adjusted to change the construct stiffness. Although in general an external fixator may provide less rigid fixation than internal fixation, its capacity for adjustment in stiffness is more advantageous in certain fractures.

Biomechanics of pin-to-bar external fixator

A pin-to-bar external fixator has three components:
- *Pins*: These are passed through the skin and fixed into the bone. There are two types of pins:
  - Half-pins emerge on one side of the limb.
  - Trans-fixation pins come through both sides of the limb.

    The bending and torsional stiffness of a pin are proportional to its radius to the fourth power. Therefore, in comparison to a 4 mm diameter pin, a 5 mm diameter pin is about one and a half times stiffer, and a 6 mm diameter pin is about five times stiffer. A stiffer pin places less stress at the bone–pin interface. However, pinholes greater than one-third of bone diameter dramatically increase the risk of fracture due to the stress raiser effect. This limits the pin size that can be used in a particular bone.

    Pins also come in a variety of profiles and thread section designs. These mainly affect the pins' purchase in the bone. The main types are discussed in the next section:
- *Bars*: These form the frame of the fixator and stabilise the fracture by spanning it between pins. Modern bars are made from carbon fibre, so are radiolucent and lightweight and still adequately stiff. The stiffness of a bar is also proportional to its radius to the fourth power.
- *Clamps*: These connect a pin to bar or a bar to bar. The clamps must securely hold the two components to maintain stiffness of the external fixator. However, they inevitably lose some grip with time, and require re-tightening periodically (Table 12.5).

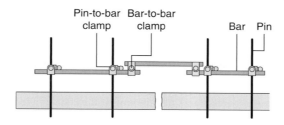

Fig. 12.33 A pin-to-bar external fixator has three components: pins, bars and clamps. A pin is technically a screw that protrudes out of the skin. It is the least stiff of the three components. The weakest point within the pin is the thread–shank junction. A bar stabilises the fracture between the pins. A simple pin-to-bar clamp connects one pin to bar, whereas a modular pin-to-bar clamp connects multiple pins to bar. An assembled externally fixator is a fixed angle device.

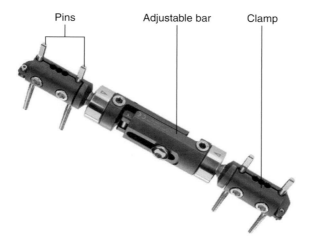

Fig. 12.34 A 'monobody' external fixator is a type of pin-to-bar external fixator, which consists of pre-assembled combined unit of clamps and bar. It has considerable inherent stiffness due to its bulky and rigid design. The pins are inserted into the bone fragments as normal and then the monobody external fixator is applied as a whole. The external fixator can be adjusted as required to facilitate fracture reduction. It is available in variable sizes for application to different bones. (Image is reproduced with permission of Orthofix.)

Table 12.5. **Guidelines on suitable pin diameter for different bones on the principle that pin diameter should not exceed a third of the diameter of the bone**

Bone	Pin diameter (mm)
Humerus	5/ 6
Radius and ulna	4
Bones in the hand	3
Femur	5/6
Tibia	5/6
Bones in the foot	3

External fixation II

Biomechanics of bone–frame construct

Bone–pin interface

The pins are inserted into bones in the 'safe zones' of the limbs to prevent injury to important soft tissue structures, e.g. nerves and arteries. The bone–pin interface is central to stability of the construct. The two main complications of an external fixator are infection and loosening at the bone–pin interface. The pin diameter is the main determinant of bone–pin interface stability. A pin with too small a diameter experiences excessive micromotion at the interface, which can lead to infection and/or fixation failure. However, the pin diameter must also not exceed one-third of the bone diameter to minimise the risk of pinhole-induced fracture.

A hydroxyapatite coating of pin threads improves pin purchase with time. Pins with conical (tapered) threads are radially pre-loaded and also maintain better purchase in bone over time. These especially 'resistant' pins are usually necessary when an external fixator is needed to definitively fix a fracture, and therefore are applied for a prolonged period of time.

Spatial configuration

External fixators can be assembled into a variety of constructs. Implant position and orientation with respect to the bone determine bone–frame stiffness:

Position of implants with respect to bone.

- Increasing the number of pins in each bone fragment distributes load over more supports and increases construct stiffness. However, this also increases the risk of infection at the bone–pin interface. Therefore, as a compromise, usually two pins are inserted in each bone segment.
- The ideal arrangement of pins in bone fragments is for the first to be close to the fracture and for the second to be as far away from the fracture as possible. This 'near–near, far–far' pin arrangement provides maximum 'control' of bone fragment and improves construct stiffness.
- The closer the bar is to the bone, the more stable the construct.
- An additional bar between the same set of pins further increases stiffness. The two bars should be arranged so that one is close to bone and the other further away from it. This 'near–near, far–far' bar arrangement further enhances construct stiffness.

Orientation of implants with respect to bone.

- External fixators are classified as unilateral and bilateral. A unilateral frame encircles up to 90° arc of area around the limb, and a bilateral frame encircles more than 90° of the limb. Both types of frames are divided further into uniplanar and biplanar. A uniplanar frame has all the pins in one plane, and a biplanar frame typically has pins at 90° to each other.
- A biplanar frame is much more stable than a uniplanar frame. It controls bending in different planes and provides high resistance against torsion. A uniplanar frame provides the most stability to the fracture when applied in the plane of bending forces.
- A triangular (also known as delta) configuration is the most stable of all the shapes.

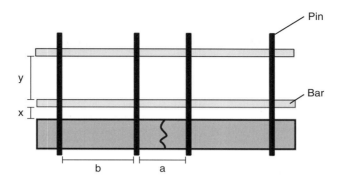

Fig. 12.35 The stiffness of a bone–frame construct is improved when pins and bars are applied in the 'near–near, far–far' arrangement. In other words, shorter distances a and x and longer distances b and y lead to a stiffer construct. However, the rigidity of fixation also depends on fracture pattern, accuracy of fracture reduction and the amount of external loading. It is imperative that the fracture is appropriately reduced to achieve adequate construct stability.

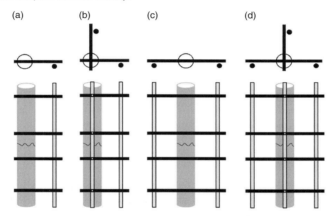

Fig. 12.36 The four main spatial configurations of pin-to-bar external fixator. Bilateral configurations are rarely used nowadays.

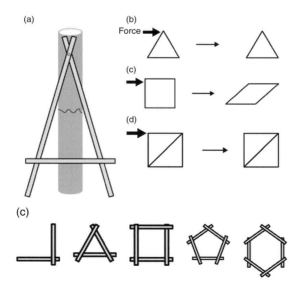

Fig. 12.37 Pin–bar–bar external fixators are commonly assembled into a 'delta' (Δ) frame. A triangle is inherently a very stable geometric shape because it is not possible to distort a triangle without distorting the actual beams. On the other hand, a square can be distorted to form a parallelogram, and therefore has less structural strength. This deformation pattern is also seen in other shapes. However, adding crossbars to these shapes to form triangles within them significantly increase their rigidity.

External fixation III

A ring external fixator provides three-dimensional stability to bone. It allows axial loading but inhibits translational and bending deflections.

Biomechanics of ring external fixator

The basic components of a ring external fixator are as follows:

- *Wires*: Thin wires of typically 1.8 mm diameter are passed across the bone to emerge on both sides of the bone. There are two types of wires.
  - Plain wires act as simple supports for the frame.
  - 'Stopper wires' have an embedded small bead (olive). These wires have two main functions. The olive in the wire can be used to help in fracture reduction by pulling a bone fragment in the required direction. The stopper wires also provide greater fixation stability by preventing undue motion.
- *Pins*: Half pins are also utilised in the circular frame construct.
- *Rings*: There are three types of rings: full (closed), partial (open) and arches. Ring properties have a significant effect on frame stability.
  - Full ring constructs are stiffer than partial ring constructs. Partial rings are applied around the joints, where full rings would prevent normal limb function or positioning.
  - Wider and thicker rings are stiffer as components, but smaller diameter rings provide a stiffer overall construct than larger diameter rings. Different diameter rings may be required within the same frame to conform to the contour of the limb.
- *Rods*: Threaded rods connect different rings.
- *Nuts and bolts*: These are used to secure the other components together.
- *Hinges and motors*: These are incorporated if controlled motion is required between different segments of the frame.

All these components are usually made of stainless steel.

Biomechanics of bone–frame construct

A number of factors determine the stiffness of bone–frame construct. The key factors are discussed below:

- Wires are inserted in pairs in bone segments. The optimal angle between wires for equal stability in all planes is 60°–90°. Stopper wires provide greater stability than plain wires when the angle between the wires is very small.
- Wires are typically tensioned to 90 kg. Paired wires must be tensioned simultaneously, as sequential tightening affects the tension in the first wire as the second wire is tensioned.
- A block of multiple rings connected together is much stiffer than a single ring. Stiffness of a multiple-ring block increases with the number of connecting rods. Therefore, a bone segment should ideally be stabilised with a ring block consisting of two rings, each with two points of fixation to bone and connected to each other with four rods.
- The construct stability is not significantly affected if the bone is not in the centre of the ring.

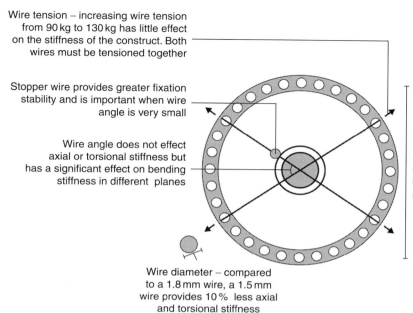

Wire tension – increasing wire tension from 90 kg to 130 kg has little effect on the stiffness of the construct. Both wires must be tensioned together

Stopper wire provides greater fixation stability and is important when wire angle is very small

Wire angle does not effect axial or torsional stiffness but has a significant effect on bending stiffness in different planes

Ring diameter determines wire length. Ring diameter has the greater effect on axial stiffness of construct. A 2 cm change in ring diameter changes construct stiffness by 15%

Wire diameter – compared to a 1.8 mm wire, a 1.5 mm wire provides 10% less axial and torsional stiffness

Fig. 12.38 The key factors that affect the stiffness of a bone–frame construct.

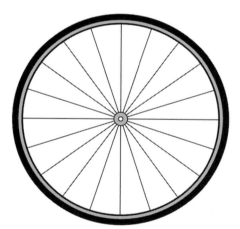

Fig. 12.39 The most essential element of a ring fixator is the tension in the wires. Equally tensioned wires support the ring of the frame in the same way as equally tensioned spokes of the wheel of a bicycle support the wheel ring. In both cases, the tension in the wires constantly *pulls* the ring together, which generates stiffness in the construct and maintains the overall shape. This allows the construct to be light and rigid.

Mechanics of trauma meeting

The trauma meeting is an integral part of orthopaedic practice. It focuses on the clinical application of biomechanics in the context of the trauma patient. There is no 'one size fits all' approach to fracture management, but biomechanical principles apply whichever treatment modality is used.

The management of a trauma patient depends on a number of factors:
- patient factors, e.g. co-morbidities, lifestyle and functional demands
- the nature of the injury, e.g. the fracture pattern, soft tissue involvement, neurovascular status and other associated injuries
- surgical factors, e.g. local expertise and surgeon's preference of treatment.

It is therefore often said in orthopaedics that the management of a fracture depends on the 'personality' of the patient, 'personality' of the fracture and 'personality' of the surgeon.

The aim of this chapter is to highlight biomechanical aspects of different treatment modalities in relation to specific fractures. It is not intended to focus on fracture classifications, on surgical technique or to provide an extensive clinical review of the outcome of treatments. Instead, the chapter focuses on biomechanical interactions between specific fractures and fixation techniques. It therefore illustrates the approach to comparing and contrasting different techniques used in the management of a family of fractures. In order to keep the discussions simple and manageable, key characteristics of implants and general trends in management are presented, and the finer points and controversies have been left out intentionally.

The aphorism 'a fracture is a soft tissue injury that happens to involve a broken bone' emphasises the importance of attention to soft tissues in any type of fracture treatment. Therefore, although the following sections evaluate different techniques mainly in relation to the fracture, the impact of the techniques on the soft tissues is also of paramount importance, and can be the determining factor in treatment selection (Table 13.1).

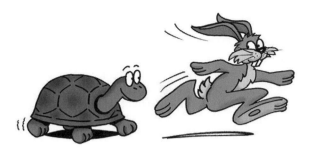

Fig. 13.1 It is usually a race between fracture healing and failure of fracture fixation. This is because the fixation device withstands all or some of the applied load until the fracture is fully united. Therefore, the fixation device could eventually experience fatigue failure if the fracture does not unite. On the other hand, once the fracture is fully united, the fixation device is superfluous.

Table 13.1. **Trauma meeting: clinical perspective**

A trauma meeting is typically held at the beginning of each day to discuss all new acute patient admissions, review the status of all trauma patients awaiting a surgical procedure, and discuss the management of any other specific patient. The preliminary order of 'trauma list' (i.e. operating list for patients with an acute injury) is usually also confirmed in the trauma meeting. It is a multi-disciplinary meeting that is typically attended by:

- members of the following teams: orthopaedics, orthogeriatrics and anaesthetics and/or staff from theatre department, e.g. scrub nurse or operating department practitioner
- trauma coordinator/ bed manager
- members of the ward staff and physiotherapy and occupational therapy teams looking after trauma patients
- staff involved in research.
- doctors from other specialties, e.g. emergency medicine, and students of the medical, nursing and allied specialties may also attend the trauma meeting.
- representatives from implant companies may also attend the meeting to learn about the upcoming operations and surgical equipment requirements.

The meeting is usually chaired by the on-call orthopaedic consultant. The junior members of the orthopaedic team present each patient and the case is then discussed. The meeting serves a number of functions, including patient handover, education and training, and research and audit.

Fractures of the middle third of clavicle

The clavicle is an S-shaped long bone that acts as a strut between the sternum and shoulder. In mechanics, a strut keeps two other components apart and resists compressive forces transmitted between them. Similarly, the clavicle lateralises the shoulder and transmits compressive forces from the upper limb to the trunk. In addition to these forces, the clavicle is also subjected to significant forces from the attached muscles.

The middle third of the clavicle has the smallest cross-sectional area, and is therefore least stiff. In addition, the ends of the clavicle are relatively stabilised by their respective articulations. As a result, the middle third of the clavicle is most prone to failure, and approximately 80% of clavicular fractures occur in this section. In the past, these fractures were considered best managed non-operatively, as almost all of these united with conservative measures. However, although the overall union rate of clavicular fractures is about 95%, the union rate in displaced fractures is approximately 85%; with the non-united fractures being quite troublesome. In addition, clavicular fractures healed in displaced position (mal-union) are also more likely to lead to problems such as residual pain and poor shoulder posture and function. Therefore, more recently there has been a shift towards surgically stabilising displaced clavicular fractures.

The mainstay treatment for most clavicular fractures is still conservative management. This usually entails application of a supportive sling or a figure-of-eight bandage; both forms of support are equally effective. The support is discarded when there is no significant motion between fracture fragments and the fracture is pain free.

Surgical treatment is considered when the fracture is shortened by >2 cm or when the fragments are displaced >100%. Other indications for surgical intervention include open fractures/ compromise of the overlying skin, neurovascular injury and floating shoulder. Displaced fractures are usually caused by high-energy injuries, and are more likely to have the associated indications for fixations.

The two primary techniques for fixing the clavicle are plate and intramedullary pin fixation. These techniques were associated previously with relatively high rates of implant-related complications, which was another reason for placing more emphasis on conservative management. However, improvements in surgical technique and design of implants have reduced these issues significantly.

Plate fixation is the more popular method for surgically stabilising a clavicular fracture. The modern plates have a low profile and may be used in locking mode to achieve high construct stability. However, a meticulous surgical technique is required to avoid injury to the vital structures in close association with the under-surface of the clavicle, e.g. the neurovascular structures and the lung. Intramedullary pin fixation allows the fragments to collapse and come together more naturally. The technique involves minimum soft tissue dissection, and the hardware is easily removed after the fracture is healed. For these reasons, intramedullary pin fixation is considered to be particularly useful for fixing clavicular fractures in children.

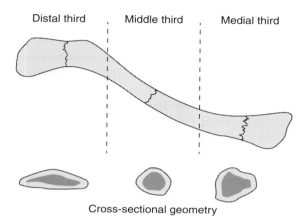

Cross-sectional geometry

Fig. 13.2 The middle third of the clavicle has the smallest cross-sectional area, and is relatively unsupported compared with the ends of the clavicle. It is therefore most prone to failure, and approximately 80% of clavicular fractures occur in this section.

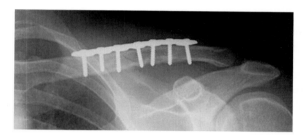

Fig. 13.3 Plate fixation allows for accurate reduction and absolute stability of clavicular fracture.

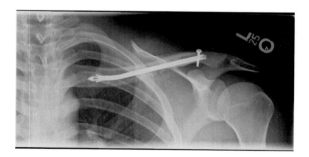

Fig. 13.4 Intramedullary pin fixation provides relative stability to clavicular fracture. The pin may be inserted antegrade or retrograde. It provides limited rotational stability. (Image courtesy of Sonoma.)

Fractures of the proximal humerus

Fractures of the proximal humerus are classified according to the number of parts to the fracture. The proximal humerus is considered to have four main parts: humeral head, shaft and greater and lesser tuberosities. A part is considered to be displaced if it is separated >1 cm or angulated >45°. Therefore, the proximal humerus can sustain a fracture of between one to four parts; the one-part fracture comprising 'undisplaced' fragments. The severity of the fracture, and the risk of avascular necrosis of humeral head, increases with the number of parts. Other factors associated with increased risk of avascular necrosis of humeral head are head-split fractures; loss of medial hinge, i.e. medial support to the humeral head; and fracture dislocations.

The goals of treatment are to maximise shoulder function and minimise pain. A number of additional factors need to be considered in deciding the appropriate treatment, e.g. bone quality and patient's age, functional level and co-morbidities. Approximately 85% of proximal humerus fractures are undisplaced or minimally displaced, i.e. consist of one part, and can be managed conservatively. Surgical intervention is generally required only if there is significant displacement between fragments or if there is an increased risk of avascular necrosis of humeral head. The two common surgical treatments for proximal humeral fractures are open reduction and internal fixation, and shoulder arthroplasty.

Open reduction and internal fixation

The principles of fixing displaced fractures are as follows:
- The head and shaft must be aligned correctly. There should be sufficient stability to allow early mobilisation.
- The tuberosities must be repositioned anatomically to balance the forces produced by the rotator cuff muscles.

The tuberosities can be re-attached using trans-osseus sutures, or anchors in a tension-band configuration. A locking compression plate is commonly used to stabilise multi-fragmented fractures. The locking plate transfers the entire load from humeral head to shaft whilst the fracture is healing, and if the fracture develops non-union (pseudoarthrosis), the plate eventually breaks due to fatigue failure.

Shoulder arthroplasty

Shoulder arthroplasty is generally considered when the fracture is not amenable to fixation, or for a three- or four-part fracture in the older osteoporotic patient. In general, there is a greater emphasis for fixing any type of fracture in the young patient and a lower threshold for shoulder replacement in the older patient. Other considerations that influence the management are the degree of underlying arthritis and integrity of the rotator cuff. The standard form of shoulder arthroplasty for proximal humerus fractures is hemiarthroplasty, and the reversed shoulder replacement is considered when there is rotator cuff deficiency or if there is a concern about realigning the tuberosities, e.g. due to severe comminution (also see pages 134–135) (Table 13.2).

(a)   (b)

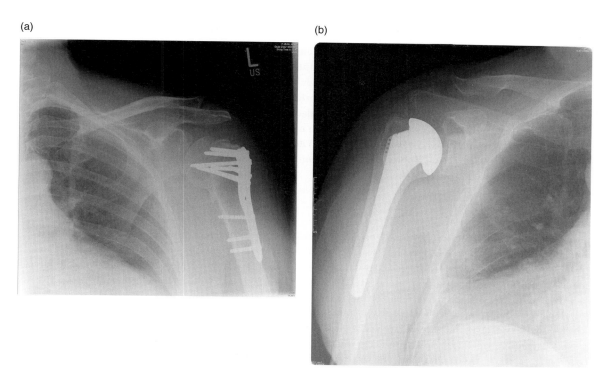

Fig. 13.5 The two common surgical treatments for proximal humeral fractures are open reduction and internal fixation, and shoulder arthroplasty. A locking compression plate is commonly used to stabilise multi-fragmented fractures. However, it is associated with high rates of complications, such as intra-articular penetration of screws, screw loosening, mal-union, non-union and avascular necrosis of humeral head. Most of these complications are considered to be related to surgical technique. The risk of fixation failure is higher in three- and four-part fractures. Therefore, there is controversy over the best management option, in terms of fixation or shoulder replacement, for these fractures in the older person. (Radiograph (b) courtesy of Arthrex.)

Table 13.2. General trends in management of the four types of proximal humerus fractures in patients of different age groups

Number of parts to the proximal humerus fracture	Age group		
	Under 50 years	50–70 years	Over 70 years
1	Conservative	Conservative	Conservative
2	ORIF	ORIF	Conservative/ ORIF**
3	ORIF	ORIF/ Shoulder replacement*	Conservative/ ORIF/ Shoulder replacement**
4	ORIF	ORIF/ Shoulder replacement*	Conservative/ ORIF/ Shoulder replacement**

* Shoulder replacement is usually considered for head-split fractures and for fracture dislocations, i.e. when there is a higher risk of avascular necrosis.
** The treatment option is matched to the patient's functional requirements and general health.

Fractures of the mid-shaft of humerus

Fractures of the mid-shaft of humerus can be managed conservatively with a functional brace in up to 90% of cases. A functional brace is a splint that fully encompasses the injured segment of the limb, but does not impede the motion of the adjacent joints. Fracture stability is achieved through hydraulic compression forces of the muscles surrounding the fracture. The humerus can tolerate up to 3 cm of shortening, 20° of anteroposterior angulation and 30° varus–valgus angulation, due to the mobility afforded by the adjacent shoulder and elbow joints.

Indications for surgical treatment include: polytrauma; open fractures; segmental or other ipsilateral fractures; pathological fractures; and failed conservative treatment. Fractures with associated neurovascular injury are generally also best managed with surgery. The two main methods of operative fixation of humeral shaft fractures are intramedullary (IM) nailing and plate fixation.

Intramedullary nailing

IM nails can be divided into two groups of design: interlocking and 'bio' nails. An interlocking nail is stabilised proximally and distally with interlocking bolts. A 'bio' nail is stabilised at the near end with interlocking bolts and at the far end with an alternative locking mechanism, e.g. manual expansion or deployment of divergent rods. Both types of nails can be inserted antegrade or retrograde. When the interlocking nail is inserted antegrade, there is a risk of iatrogenic injury to neurovascular structures during distal locking. The bio nail reduces the risk of this complication; however, fixation stability is reduced when compared with the interlocking nail. Therefore, the interlocking nail usually provides adequate stability, regardless of direction of insertion in relation to fracture location. However, the stability of fixation with 'bio' nail is better if the interlocking bolts at the near end of the nail are closer to the fracture site. Therefore, a 'bio' nail should ideally be inserted antegrade if the fracture is in the proximal half of the humerus and retrograde if the fracture is in the distal half of the humerus.

Plate fixation

This is the gold standard for surgical fixation of humeral shaft fractures. Fracture configuration dictates the mode in which the plate is applied. A transverse fracture can be fixed with direct compression plating; a short oblique or a spiral fracture may be stabilised with lag screws with the plate applied in neutralisation mode; and, in comminuted fractures, the plate is applied in bridging mode. The use of locking plates is advantageous in the setting of poor bone quality but not in fracture comminution *per se*. There should ideally be a minimum of six cortices' fixation on either side of the fracture (Table 13.3).

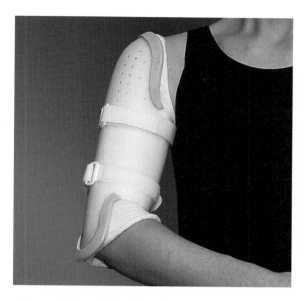

Fig. 13.6 The functional brace works by creating a cylinder of set volume around the limb. When the muscles contract, their attempted increase in size produces a hydraulic compressive force that stabilises the fracture. Therefore, a functional brace stabilises, but does not immobilise, the fracture. Although the fracture ends are relatively mobile, they return to the original position because the compressive force is uniformly distributed within the cylinder. The principle of soft tissue containment does not depend on the stiffness of the bracing material, but instead on the set volume of the cylinder formed. (Image courtesy of Patterson Medical Ltd.)

Table 13.3. Clinical and biomechanical considerations in intramedullary and plate fixation of humoral shaft fractures

	Intramedullary nailing	Plate fixation
Advantages	The IM nail is a load-sharing implant. Its placement in the medullary canal aligns it with mechanical axis of the bone, and therefore it is subjected to lower bending stresses. It requires smaller surgical incisions, and involves less soft tissue stripping.	Plate fixation can be performed through a variety of surgical approaches. The neurovascular structures, especially the radial nerve, are directly visualised and their integrity confirmed. It is associated with much lower rates of fracture non-union than IM nailing.
Limitations	There is a high incidence of 'insertion site' morbidity. The antegrade technique is associated with shoulder complications, such as rotator cuff dysfunction, frozen shoulder and subacromial impingement syndrome. The retrograde technique is associated with iatrogenic fractures. 'Bio' nails have a high secondary complication rate due to insufficient rotational stability. IM nailing is contraindicated in open fractures and in fractures associated with neurological deficit.	This is a load-bearing implant, and can theoretically lead to stress-shielding osteopenia. Complication rate ranges from 3% to 13%. The range of complications is similar to those occurring in plate fixation of other fractures, e.g. infection, mal-union, non-union and neurovascular injury. It is important to document where the radial nerve crosses the plate – this is useful in future surgery.

Intra-articular fractures of distal humerus

The standard management for intra-articular fractures of distal humerus is open reduction and internal fixation with plates and screws. The principles of fixation are: anatomic reduction of articular fragments; restoration of normal alignment between humeral shaft and distal fragments; and provision of a stable construct to allow for early, active elbow mobilisation. The distal humerus consists of distinct medial and lateral columns. The fixation is more stable when both columns are plated than when only one column is plated. In the double-plating technique, the plates can be applied perpendicular or parallel to each other. In both methods, the fracture is anatomically reduced, and is often temporarily stabilised with k-wires, before the application of plates.

The perpendicular plate configuration is the traditional approach to two-column plate fixation. It involves the application of one plate to the medial supracondylar ridge of the humerus and the other plate to the posterolateral aspect of the lateral side of the humerus. The parallel plate configuration is a comparatively new concept in which the plates are applied along the medial and lateral supracondylar ridges. The plates used in both configurations are usually the locking type and pre-contoured. The locking plates provide a more stable fixation than non-locking plates in poor-quality bone or when the fracture is highly comminuted.

From a biomechanical perspective, the parallel plate configuration provides a significantly stiffer and stronger fixation than the perpendicular plate configuration. This is due to a combination of factors. Firstly, there are generally more screws fixing the fracture in the parallel plate configuration, and the screws are usually also longer, as they are all applied across the medio-lateral width of the humerus. Secondly, according to the principle of area moment of inertia, parallel plating provides a higher resistance to bending in the antero-posterior direction, which is the main type of load acting at the fracture due to flexion–extension motion of the adjacent elbow joint. Thirdly, the overall construct of parallel plate fixation locks the medial and lateral columns together in the form of an arch, which is an inherently stable arrangement.

However, from a clinical perspective, both methods stabilise the fracture adequately to achieve fracture union. As perpendicular plate configuration has been used for longer, a number of clinical studies are available to show the long-term results of this method of fixation. These studies indicate that this technique provides satisfactory outcome with long-term follow-up. On the other hand, parallel plate configuration does not have such a long clinical track record, but the available data indicate that this technique also provides comparable clinical results.

Finally, from a surgical perspective, there are some suggestions that plate application to the lateral condylar ridge can be technically difficult, and that parallel plate configuration is associated with more extensive subperiosteal elevation, which can increase the risk of delayed union and non-union.

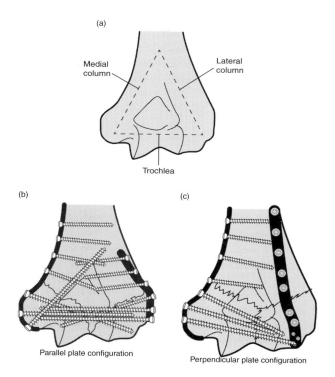

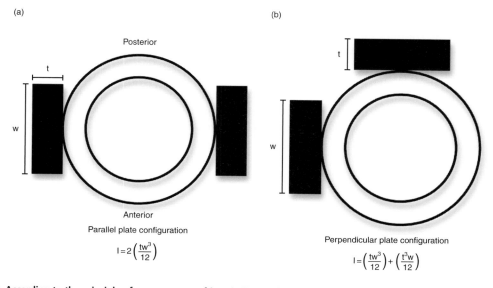

Fig. 13.7 The distal humerus relies on a triangular construct for stability. (a) The walls of the triangle are formed by medial and lateral columns and the trochlea. Intra-articular fractures of distal humerus affect all three walls. The standard management for these fractures is open reduction and internal fixation with plates and screws. In the double-plating technique, the plates can be applied perpendicular or parallel to each other. (b) Parallel plate configuration provides significantly stiffer and stronger fixation than (c) perpendicular plate configuration.

Parallel plate configuration

$$I = 2\left(\frac{tw^3}{12}\right)$$

Perpendicular plate configuration

$$I = \left(\frac{tw^3}{12}\right) + \left(\frac{t^3w}{12}\right)$$

Fig. 13.8 According to the principle of area moment of inertia (I), parallel plate configuration (a) provides a higher resistance to bending in the antero-posterior direction than (b) in the perpendicular plate configuration (see pages 56–57 footnotes). Figures (a) and (b) show models of the axial views of the distal humerus with plates applied.

Distal radius fractures

These are amongst the commonest bone fractures. The mode of treatment depends on the fracture configuration and on the functional demands of the patient. The majority of these fractures are managed satisfactorily with closed reduction and cast treatment. However, a small proportion may require percutaneous k-wire fixation or open reduction and internal fixation.

Percutaneous k-wire fixation

This is undertaken in cases where the fracture has enough inherent stability to be managed in a cast, but either it cannot be reduced fully with manipulation or it is considered to require further support to maintain satisfactory alignment until union. This judgement is usually made at the time of closed reduction of the fracture, although the fracture pattern may provide an indication of fracture stability beforehand. Different types of fractures require different numbers of stabilising k-wires, which are applied in various configurations based on the fracture pattern. The most common configuration consists of a 'dorsal' wire and a 'radial styloid' wire. The patient is managed in a cast and the wires are usually removed at 6 weeks. The results of k-wire fixation are generally better in younger patients than in older patients, as k-wires maintain a better hold in normal bone than in osteoporotic bone.

Kapandji k-wiring technique

This technique is typically used to reduce and stabilise an extra-articular distal radius fracture. It involves percutaneously inserting a k-wire through the fracture site. Then, the near end of the k-wire is arced towards the distal fragment. This manoeuvre levers the distal fragment into the reduced position. Once an adequate position is achieved, the k-wire is driven through the far cortex to achieve stability. The k-wire does not fix the distal fragment, but instead provides buttress support.

Open reduction and internal fixation

The threshold in terms of fracture characteristics for consideration of open reduction and internal fixation includes radial shortening > 3 cm, dorsal tilt >10° or an intra-articular step >2 mm after attempted closed reduction. This is also indicated in fractures that may initially be satisfactorily reduced, but have a high risk of displacement due to the basic fracture pattern. Fractures with associated neurovascular injury are generally also best managed with surgery.

There has been a transformation in the internal fixation technique over time. In the past, dorsal plating was the most popular method. As most distal radius fractures are displaced dorsally, this worked on the principle of buttressing the fragments to prevent fracture displacement. However, the site of plate application – under the extensor compartments of the wrist – was a compromise, and dorsal plating was associated with tendonitis and rupture of extensor tendons. Still, this was the most mechanically sound method of fracture fixation. The emergence of fixed-angle volar locking plate stimulated interest in volar plating, and this has now become the most commonly used internal fixation technique.

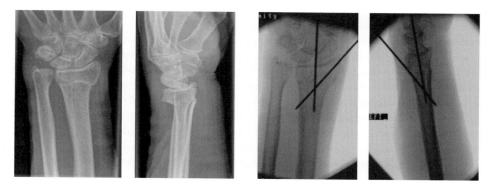

Fig. 13.9 An example of the use of k-wires to stabilise a distal radius fracture. Here, one dorsal and one radial styloid wire are adequate to provide stable, three-dimensional fixation. The dorsal k-wire has been applied with the Kapandji tehnique. The principles of k-wire fixation discussed on pages 166–167 have also been applied.

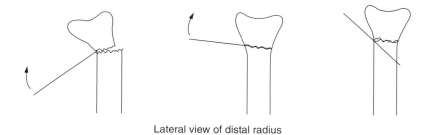

Lateral view of distal radius

Fig. 13.10 Kapandji k-wiring technique is typically used to reduce and stabilise an extra-articular distal radius fracture.

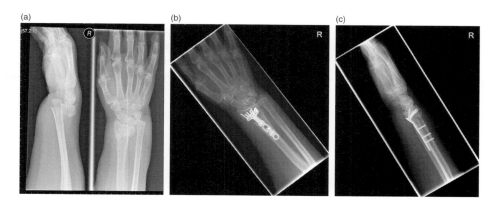

Fig. 13.11 Open reduction and internal fixation enables more accurate fracture reduction and provides greater stability. The most commonly used internal fixation technique is volar plating. This technique is effective because the distal screws holding the bone fragments (which are often very comminuted) are fastened into the locking plate and therefore are prevented from backing out. The construct has very high stability, despite relatively poor bone quality and low intrinsic fracture stability.

Intertrochanteric fractures of the proximal femur

An intertrochanteric fracture divides the proximal femur into two main parts: one consisting of femoral head and neck and the other consisting of femoral shaft. These main parts may be fragmented even further, e.g. a typical four-part fracture consists of femoral head and neck, femoral shaft, greater trochanter and lesser trochanter fragments. The main fracture line usually runs obliquely from the greater trochanter to the lesser trochanter. However, in a 'reverse oblique' fracture, the main fracture line runs from intertrochanteric region distally to lateral femoral cortex. In addition, in a 'subtrochanteric' fracture, the main fracture line extends distal to the lesser trochanter. The intertrochanteric fracture does not affect the blood supply to the femoral head and is therefore suitable for fixation. However, different types of intertrochanteric fractures have different intrinsic fracture stability.

The two implants commonly used for treatment of intertrochanteric fractures are dynamic hip screw (DHS) and IM nail. The goal of fixation is to achieve a construct sufficiently stable to allow immediate full weight-bearing and rehabilitation. Both implants utilise a cancellous lag screw to stabilise the femoral head. The lag screw has a purchase in the femoral head but not in the shaft; therefore, weight-bearing leads to a directed sliding of the femoral head, which produces compression at the fracture site. The two devices differ in how the lag screw is connected to the femoral shaft.

Dynamic hip screw

This consists of a plate with an extension (barrel) that slides over the lag screw. The plate is fixed to the femoral shaft with a number of screws. The plate is not secured mechanically to the lag screw; therefore, during weight-bearing the lag screw slides down within the barrel of the plate, allowing the femoral head to slide down as well, thereby compressing the fracture. Weight-bearing also produces a bending moment, which acts to displace the fracture. The plate–lag screw connection prevents the lag screw from bending, and the screws fixing the plate to the femoral shaft prevent the plate from bending.

Intramedullary nail

In this setting, an IM nail is also referred to as a 'cephalomedullary' implant. The lag screw is inserted *after* the placement of IM nail. The lag screw may be free to slide through the nail, or be fixed in its position; weight-bearing allows the femoral head to slide down and compress the fracture in both cases. The nail is fixed to the femoral shaft with the distal screw(s). Again, the bending moment is resisted by the lag screw–IM nail construct. There is a choice of short or long IM nail, depending on the fracture configuration and/or whether there is a need to support the whole bone.

In both methods, a further 'derotational' screw may be used to provide additional rotational stability to the fracture.

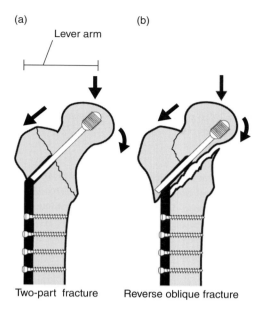

Two-part fracture   Reverse oblique fracture

Fig. 13.12 Mechanics of intertrochanteric fracture fixation with dynamic hip screw. The DHS is a load-bearing implant. Bending stiffness of DHS plate is proportional to its thickness to the third power. The bending moment produced is greater than in IM nail fixation, as there is a longer lever arm between the plate and applied force. (a) The DHS is ideal for use in intertrochanteric fractures with stable configurations. The fracture becomes progressively less stable with increasing number of parts, requiring more support from the implant. (b) The reverse oblique and subtrochanteric fractures are inherently unstable as there is a loss of 'lateral buttress' support; so with DHS fixation, the proximal fragments continue to slide down unstopped, leading to medial relative displacement of the femoral shaft.

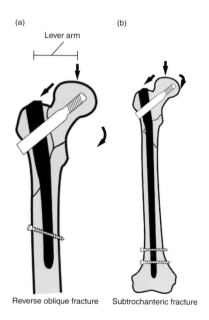

Reverse oblique fracture   Subtrochanteric fracture

Fig. 13.13 Mechanics of intertrochanteric fracture fixation with an intramedullary nail. The IM nail is a load-sharing implant. It provides a more stable fixation than the DHS for two main reasons: the IM nail is a stiffer implant than DHS because its bending stiffness is proportional to its radius to the fourth power; and the bending moment produced is less than in DHS fixation, as the IM nail takes up a more medial position and therefore the lever arm between the implant and applied force is shorter. However, clinically, IM nail has a clear advantage over the DHS in (a) reverse oblique and (b) subtrochanteric fracture configurations. In these fractures, the shaft of IM nail forms the lateral buttress and limits the displacement of the proximal fragments. A long IM nail may be required for subtrochanteric fractures or if there is a need to support the whole bone prophylactically.

Fractures of distal third of tibia

Fractures of distal third of tibia vary in pattern from the simple extra-articular type to those with intra-articular tibial plafond extension and more severe pilon fractures. These fractures can be managed with a number of different methods. Each method has advantages and limitations, and currently there is no consensus on the most appropriate method for treating these fractures. This section considers the biomechanical issues related to fixation of an isolated, simple extra-articluar fracture of distal third of tibia with two common techniques: IM nailing and plate fixation.

Intramedullary nailing

IM nailing is considered to be the treatment of choice for most fractures of the mid-diaphysis of tibia. It is also used for fixing fractures of the distal third of tibia. However, the biomechanical issues in IM nail fixation of the two types of fractures are quite different. In the mid-diaphyseal fracture, the bone–implant construct is inherently stable, as the tubular profile of bone in the diaphyseal region means that fracture generally needs to be quite well aligned for the nail to cross the fracture site, and so there is extensive contact between the bone and the nail. However, in the fractures of the distal third of tibia, the bone–implant construct is inherently less stable, because in the wider distal third section, there is limited direct contact between the bone and the nail. This can cause difficulty in achieving the correct alignment of fracture. The limited bone–implant contact means that most of the stability is provided by distal interlocking screws. It further means that there is increased stress on the interlocking screws (see pages 176–177), which therefore are more prone to breakage.

Plate fixation

A low profile, contoured, locking compression plate is another popular choice for fixing this fracture. Other types of plate, e.g. a dynamic compression plate or a T-plate, can also be used. The usual approach for plating is anteromedial, although an anterolateral approach is also used. The anterolateral approach has the advantage that it can also be used to fix the fibula fracture if required.

The plate can be applied with either the standard open reduction and internal fixation technique, in which the fracture is fully exposed and anatomically reduced, and the plate is applied with the aim of achieving interfragmentary compression; or with a minimally invasive plate osteosynthesis (MIPO) technique, in which the fracture is reduced closed and the plate is applied through a small incision and the screws are inserted through 'stab' incisions. The MIPO technique places emphasis on restoring the tibial mechanical axis (rather than anatomically reducing the fragments) and on protecting the soft tissues around the fracture site.

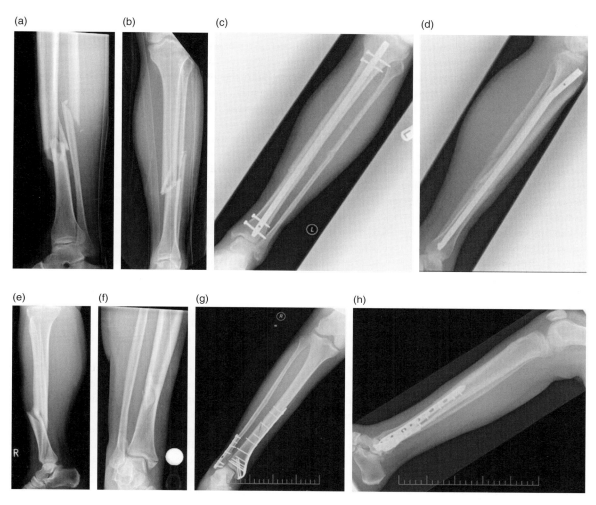

Fig. 13.14 Fractures of the distal tibia may be surgically managed with intramedullary nailing or plate fixation. It is usually not possible to use the IM nailing technique if the fracture line extends to within 5 cm of the ankle joint. Advocates of IM nailing emphasise that the reaming required before nail insertion helps to proliferate the fracture repair process and that the zone of injury is not disturbed by dissection. The plate may be applied in a number of different modes, e.g. in neutralisation, compression or bridging mode. Meta-analyses of studies comparing the outcomes of the two techniques show that IM nailing is associated with a higher risk of knee pain (because it requires surgical approach around the knee joint for nail insertion) and mal-union (as it can be difficult to achieve and maintain correct rotation of fragments with the IM nail), whereas plate fixation is associated with a higher risk of superficial wound infections. There is no difference between the techniques in time to fracture union and fracture non-union rates and other functional results.

Pilon fractures

A pilon fracture is a comminuted fracture of the distal tibia that extends into the tibial plafond. The term pilon is French for pestle, which reflects the shape of the distal tibia.

The pilon fracture typically is caused by an axial compression injury that drives the talus into the tibia. The talus is one and a half times stronger than the distal tibia, and a severe impact causes the tibial articular surface to fracture into fragments. The injury may result in damage to the articular surface of the talus. In addition, there is often also an associated distal fibula fracture.

This is a severe injury that consists of three elements: fracture comminution, disruption of the articular surface and associated soft tissue swelling. The standard treatment for this fracture is surgical fixation. It is common practice to stabilise the fracture temporarily with a pin-to-bar external fixator. The definitive surgery can then be delayed until the soft tissue swelling has settled. In the meantime, it is usually also necessary to have further imaging of the fracture, in the form of a CT scan, to plan surgery. The principles of initial management are aptly summarised as 'span, scan and plan'.

The surgical techniques for definitive fixation of pilon fracture can be divided into two groups: open reduction and internal fixation, and external fixation. The principles of both treatments are management of soft tissues, reconstruction of joint line and realignment of the mechanical axis of tibia. Open reduction and internal fixation involves direct reconstruction of tibial articular surface, bone grafting to support the reconstructed joint line, and application of a bridging plate and in certain cases buttress plate(s) as well. Depending on fracture configuration, free-standing screws may also be applied to fix specific fragments, e.g. if there is a significant fracture line in the coronal plane, a screw may be applied from anterior to posterior with the aim of 'capturing' and stabilising a large posterior fragment. The procedure is performed through as small an incision as possible to minimise injury to the soft tissue envelope.

External fixation involves closed or minimally invasive reduction of articular surface, which may be supplemented with limited internal fixation, e.g. free-standing screws, and application of an external fixator to maintain mechanical alignment until fracture heals. The external fixator utilises the principle of ligamentotaxis to provide stability. Both pin-to-bar and circular frames can be utilised, or a hybrid frame consisting of straight bars and rings may also be used. The pin-to-bar frame is usually monolateral and bridging-type, i.e. it spans across the ankle joint.

There is no consensus on the management of the associated fibula fracture. Fixing the fibula fracture can help to maintain the length and alignment of the pilon fracture. However, this involves an additional incision, which can increase the risk of wound complications.

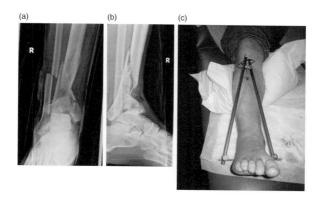

Fig. 13.15 **A pilon fracture is a comminuted fracture of the distal tibia that extends into the tibial plafond.** It is estimated that up to a quarter of these fractures are also open. A temporary external fixator commonly is applied to stabilise the fracture and allow soft tissues management before further surgery. The temporary external fixator spans the ankle joint and is usually applied in triangular configuration, i.e. as a 'delta' (Δ) frame. Depending on the reduction and stability achieved, a temporary external fixator could even be used for long-term treatment. (Image (c) is reproduced with permission of Tony Meehan.)

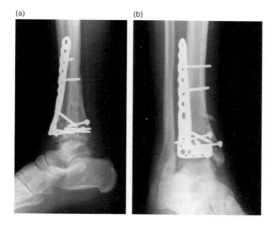

Fig. 13.16 **These radiographs show an example of a pilon fracture managed with open reduction and internal fixation.** Here, a locking plate has been applied in bridging mode.

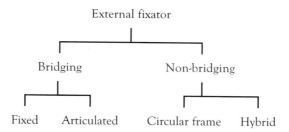

Fig. 13.17 **Classification of different external fixation constructs that can be used to manage pilon fractures.** The term 'bridging' means the same as 'spanning'.

Ankle fractures

The stability of the ankle joint is derived from congruency of the articulating surfaces and from the soft tissues, i.e. the ligaments. The treatment of ankle fractures is based on not only the fracture, but also on how it affects the stability of the joint. In ankle fractures, the term 'stability' is more often used in the context of the joint than the fracture. The two main groups of treatments for ankle fractures are conservative, and open reduction and internal fixation. The algorithm for management of ankle fractures is extensive, due to the variety in ankle fracture patterns and in treatment options in each group. The following is intended to be a simple guide to the basic principles of the two types of management.

Conservative treatment

Conservative treatment is ideal for stable ankle fractures, i.e. when the joint is stable and the talus is undisplaced. The deltoid (medial) ligament is central to maintaining joint stability in ankle fractures. It originates from the medial malleolus and inserts onto the medial aspect of the talus, and therefore prevents the talus from displacing laterally. An ankle fracture can be managed conservatively if the deltoid ligament is intact. An example of a stable ankle fracture is the isolated fracture of the lateral malleolus. However, a lateral malleolar fracture with tenderness over the medial malleolus, which suggests deltoid ligament rupture, is potentially unstable. It may still be managed conservatively (at least initially) if there is no associated lateral talar shift.

Open reduction and internal fixation

This is indicated for unstable ankle fractures, i.e. for when the ankle joint is not congruent. The examples of unstable ankle fractures include a lateral malleolar fracture with lateral talar shift and bimalleolar and trimalleolar fractures. In all these cases, the deltoid ligament is non-functional. In a trimalleolar fracture, the posterior malleolus usually only requires fixing if it is more than a third of the articular surface, and therefore is likely to affect joint stability.

These fractures may also be associated with diastasis of distal tibiofibular syndesmosis; which appears as widening of the normal space between the tibia and fibula. If the syndesmosis requires fixing, then a long screw is used to hold the fibula and tibia in the anatomical position whilst the syndesmosis heals. According to the biomechanical studies, one 3.5 mm cortical screw passed across three cortices, i.e. lateral and medial cortices of fibula and lateral cortex of tibia, about 2.5 cm above the ankle joint line is usually adequate for stability. It is important that the ankle is in dorsiflexion when the syndesmosis screw is inserted to ensure that the wider, anterior aspect of talus is engaged in the mortise, which prevents over-tightening of the screw.

Isolated fractures of the medial malleolus are also fixed routinely to restore the ankle mortise, although undisplaced medial malleolar fractures may be managed conservatively.

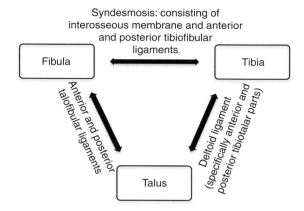

Fig. 13.18 **The ligaments are the most important soft tissues for maintaining joint stability, as there are no muscles directly acting on the talus.** Disruption of the deltoid ligament allows the talus to displace laterally. Similarly, injury to the syndesmosis leads to diastasis between the tibia and the fibula. The diastasis itself does not predispose to lateral talar shift, but it is associated invariably with deltoid ligament injury and therefore with an unstable ankle.

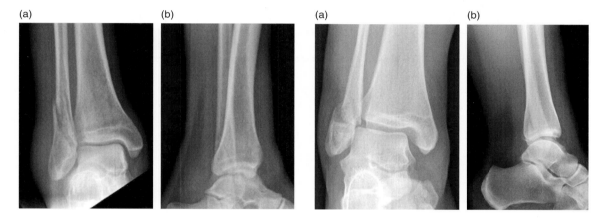

Fig. 13.19 **This is an example of a stable ankle fracture.** The deltoid ligament is intact and the talus is undisplaced.

Fig. 13.20 **This is an example of an unstable ankle fracture.** The deltoid ligament is disrupted and there is lateral talar shift.

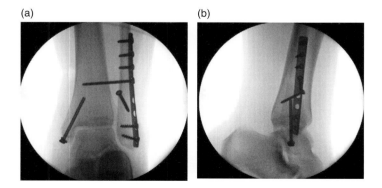

Fig. 13.21 **This is an example of a severe ankle fracture that has been internally fixed.** The lateral malleolus has been fixed with a plate applied in neutralisation mode. The medial malleolus has been fixed with two partially threaded cancellous screws, which by design are acting as lag screws. The ankle syndesmosis has also been fixed.

Further reading

Banaszkiewicz PA, Kader DF (eds) (2012). *Postgraduate Orthopaedics: The Candidate's Guide to the FRCS (Tr and Orth) Examination*. 2nd edn. Cambridge: Cambridge University Press.

Bucholz RW, Court-Brown CM, Heckman JD, Tornetta P (eds) (2009). *Rockwood and Green's Fractures in Adults*. 7th edn. Vol. 1 and 2. New York: Lippincott, Williams and Wilkins.

Burstein AH, Wright TM (1994). *Fundamentals of Orthopaedic Biomechanics*. New York: Lippincott, Williams and Wilkins.

Charnley J (1999). *The Closed Treatment of Common Fractures*. Cambridge: Cambridge University Press.

Dandy DJ, Edwards DJ (2009). *Essential Orthopaedics and Trauma*. 5th edn. London: Churchill Livingstone, Elsevier.

Denis F (1984). Spinal instability as defined by the three-column spine concept in acute spinal trauma. *Clin Orthop Relat Res*. 189: 65–76.

Gougoulias NE, Khanna A, Maffulli N (2009). History and evolution in total ankle arthroplasty. *Br Med Bull*. 89: 111–151.

Holdsworth F (1970). Fractures, dislocations and fracture–dislocations of the spine. *JBJS-A*. 52: 1534–1551.

Knahr K (ed) (2011). *Tribology in Total Hip Arthroplasty*. London: Springer.

Lucas GL, Cooke FW, Friis EA (1999). *A Primer of Biomechanics*. New York: Springer-Verlag.

Miller MD, Thompson SR, Hart J (2012). *Review of Orthopaedics*. 6th edn. Philadelphia: Saunders.

Mow VC, Huiskes R (2005). *Basic Orthopaedic Biomechanics and Mechano-biology*. 3rd edn. New York: Lippincott, Williams and Wilkins.

Nordin M, Frankel VH (2001). *Basic Biomechanics of the Musculoskeletal System*. 3rd edn. London: Lippincott, Williams and Wilkins.

Ruedi TP, Buckley RE, Moran CG (2007). *AO Principles of Fracture Management*. 2nd edn. Vol. 1 and 2. New York: Thieme.

Solomon L, Warwick D, Nayagam S (eds) (2010). *Apley's System of Orthopaedics and Fractures*. 9th edn. New York: CRC Press.

Vickerstaff JA, Miles AW, Cunningham JL (2007). A brief history of total ankle replacement and a review of the current status. *Med Eng Phys*. 29: 1056–1064.

White AP, Panjabi MM (eds) (1990). *Clinical Biomechanics of the Spine*. Philadelphia: Lippincott, Williams & Wilkins.